AF375214

TAKING CARE OF MOM

A Son's Perspective on Being A Caregiver

Jim Heath

ISPN: 979-8-9904811-0-7

Printed in the United States of America

ABOUT THE BOOK

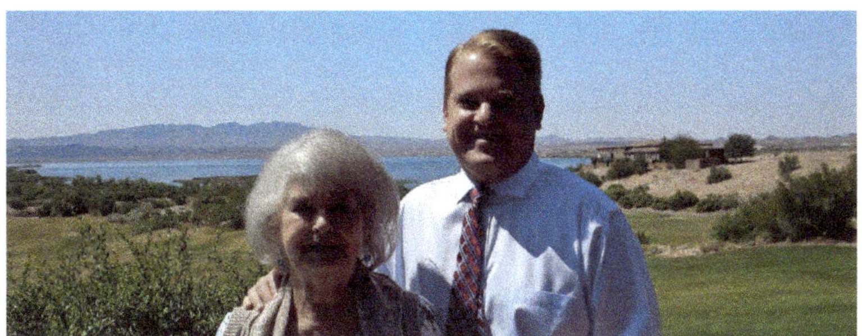

"Taking Care of Mom" is a poignant guide and companion for anyone preparing to navigate the challenging journey of saying the final goodbye to a loved one. This book explores the emotional and practical aspects of caregiving through the lens of Jim Heath, who steps into the role of caregiver for his ailing mother, Doris Heath. It delves into Jim's personal experiences, from managing daily care complexities to tackling the societal norms around gender and caregiving, all while showcasing the deep, unbreakable bond he shares with his mother.

Set against the backdrop of their rich shared history, the narrative unfolds as Jim, leaving behind his award-winning broadcasting career, transitions into the deeply intimate role of caregiver. This transformative journey is portrayed through heartfelt stories filled with love, resilience, and the profound connection between mother and son.

Through Jim's personal anecdotes, reflections, and advice, "Taking Care of Mom" provides invaluable insights into the nuanced challenges and rewards of caregiving. It addresses the stigma often associated with male caregivers and advocates for a shift in societal perspectives to recognize the compassion and strength that sons can bring to caregiving roles.

This book is crafted to resonate with readers on a deeply personal level yet remains universally relatable, emphasizing the importance of empathy, understanding, and the courage needed to embrace vulnerability. More than a mere narrative, "Taking Care of Mom" serves as a celebration of enduring love and a practical guide for those embarking on this emotionally charged farewell. It aims to foster a more inclusive, compassionate approach to caregiving, making it an essential read for anyone in a similar situation.

What They're Saying

"Taking Care of Mom" has garnered acclaim from readers and critics alike, each offering their unique insights into the profound impact of Jim Heath's narrative. Here's what they're saying:

"This is truly a beautiful and important book. So timely too. It deals with a subject people don't want to think about until they are faced with it - and it's often too late. Jim Heath's care of his mother was exemplary on every level. 'Taking Care of Mom' should be required reading for everyone." — Kaisu Fisken

"The story is at once heartwarming and heartbreaking. It is an end-of-life love story between a mother and son who face together the encroaching darkness of dementia with patience and courage. It is a roadmap for others who choose personal homes instead of nursing homes for a tender goodbye." — Marcey Forman

"A hero, serving his hero. The selfless and raw journey of caregiving. An unbreakable beautiful love story." — Kaushal Patel

"Jim's experiences are authentic and relatable to other caregivers who are going through the emotional process of helping someone they love through the transition of leaving this world behind. In particular, his observations as a male caregiver bring to the forefront a stigma perpetuated throughout time and one that policymakers, health providers, and society, in general, should give more consideration and contemplation. Jim's devotion to his family, particularly to his parents, is a testament to the powerful love they gave him throughout his lifetime. And it is an example of how love facilitates strength and comfort that is needed when dealing with the tough challenge of letting go of someone special without relinquishing their dignity." — Jo Ingles

"It took me a few days to read Jim's book; I shed many tears as it reminded me of my own father's passing. The book offers insightful suggestions and honest reflections. Doris was loved by all who knew her, and Jim is a saint. It's beautiful." — Heather Moore

"Taking Care of Mom is a must-read for anyone faced with the challenges of being a caregiver for an elderly parent. Jim Heath's raw, emotional storytelling takes readers on this journey with him as he navigates the sacrifices and realities of this difficult, yet rewarding experience, and the unbreakable bond between mother and son weathering a particularly cruel illness. Through Jim's honesty and vulnerability, we're able to glean what he learned as his mother's caregiver, a gift to anyone in a similar circumstance." — Connie Weber

This collection of reviews captures the heartfelt and transformative essence of "Taking Care of Mom," highlighting its relevance to those facing the challenges of caregiving and shedding light on the broader societal implications of gender roles in caregiving.

FOREWORD

By Kaisu Fisken, RN

I am honored to write this foreword for Jim's beautiful, life-affirming, and valuable book. I first met Jim and the beautiful Doris Heath as they embarked on their journey with palliative care. Focused on the patient, I was immediately struck by the grace, elegance, and kindness that Doris radiated. Despite being immensely troubled by her increasing memory lapses and failing physical strength, her spirit remained indomitable. I quickly became aware of the unfailing love, kindness, and commitment displayed by her primary caregiver, her son Jim. The three of us traversed a wide swath of topics as I labored to provide the education, resources, and support this challenging phase of life demanded. It truly was an honor and a privilege to be part of their journey.

Jim stood out because most primary caregivers I encountered were daughters. Here was a son who had made the immense commitment of time, energy, and effort this role demanded. I learned that Jim was a gifted writer, thinker, and newscaster. The immensity of his sacrifice is humbling.

As our population ages, and with dementia in the diagnosis for approximately 50% of people over age 80, this wealthy, vibrant country must look at changes in our care of the people we love, those that loved us first. Currently, our system is set up to send people to assisted care facilities. I cannot overemphasize the distress this causes for those who rely on routine, familiar places, and faces. It truly is heartbreaking to try and respond to lovely people who want to know "Why did they send me away?" It is as heartbreaking to respond to equally lovely people who resist this step as long as is humanly possible and want to know "Did I do the right thing?"

We must begin to divert some resources away from facilities to supports for people wanting to age in place. In other countries, professional caregivers are paid to render care in the home. Without such support, caregivers like Jim face challenges that are mentally, physically, emotionally, and spiritually daunting. It is also crucial for everyone involved in the system to recognize that these journeys are as unique as the individuals taking them. It can be rewarding, enriching, and life-affirming, expanding our minds and spirits as nothing else quite can.

There is no doubt in my mind, Jim, that the love you shared with your mother will never die. Just as others will surely encourage you after turning the final page of this book, I too urge you: keep checking that lock.

All my love,

Kaisu

Note From the Author

If you had told me a decade ago that I'd be sitting down to write a book about caregiving, I would have chuckled at the notion. The world of caregiving, particularly for men treading the delicate path of caring for their aging parents, often feels like uncharted territory, lacking in tailored guidance or resources. For the longest time, I cherished the freedom and independence of my career and bachelor lifestyle, purposefully avoiding the weighty responsibilities synonymous with parenthood. Little did I know that life had a way of weaving its unexpected threads, subtly nudging me into a realm of profound human obligation.

The turning point came when I witnessed my mother, Doris—my steadfast rock and best friend—grappling with the harsh realities of aging. As her health began to falter, I found myself thrust into a role I had never envisioned: the primary caregiver for the woman who had given me life. This experience shattered my preconceived notions of caregiving and fundamentally reshaped my sense of self.

This book represents my heartfelt attempt to navigate this transformative odyssey, serving as a guiding beacon for family caregivers, particularly sons, who may feel overlooked or unprepared for the challenges that lie ahead. It's a deeply personal exploration of my journey to confront and eventually embrace caregiving, unveiling the unexpected treasures hidden within this role. Woven within my own narrative with my mother is a broader discourse on the gender dynamics of caregiving, aimed at dispelling the stigmas surrounding male caregivers.

Amidst the peaks and valleys of my journey with my mother, I discovered the true essence of caregiving as an expression of profound love and respect. It afforded me the opportunity to repay, in some measure, the care I had once received.

With this book, I aim to share insights and wisdom gleaned from my experiences, offering more than just a roadmap—it's a testament to the transformative power of caregiving to forge deeper connections and reveal our most authentic selves. It challenges societal norms surrounding caregiving, advocating for a future where caregiving is revered as an integral aspect of our shared humanity. I want to show you that you, too, can navigate this journey with grace and resilience. Despite my initial reluctance to embrace the responsibilities of caregiving, my parents found a way to draw me into this fundamental aspect of life's journey, reshaping my understanding of love, duty, and human connection.

This narrative isn't solely mine; it's also a tribute to my mother, the most extraordinary human being I've ever known, and a reflection on the profound self-discovery that emerged from caring for her. My hope is that it serves as a guiding light for others, illuminating the profound love, sacrifice, and self-discovery inherent in the act of caregiving.

Doris Jean Heath

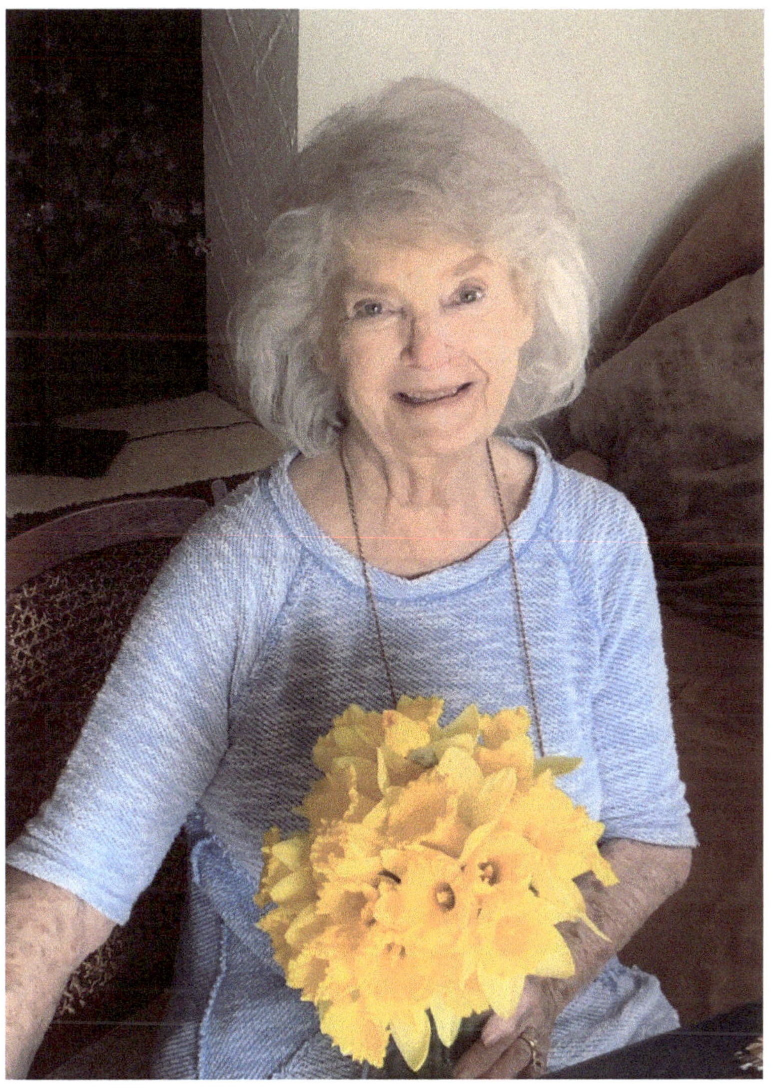

Being deeply loved by someone gives you strength, while loving someone deeply gives you courage. • Lao Tzu

Memory Keeper

In the quiet hours before dawn, in the home where I was raised, I laid in bed next to my mother. This house, once filled with the laughter and chaos of a bustling family, now echoes with the quiet passage of time and the unspoken understanding of what's to come. I've come a long way from the bright lights of the broadcasting world, where my face and voice were known to many local viewers. But here, in this moment, none of that seems to matter. What matters is her—my mother, my guiding star, who's slowly fading into the final sunset of her life.

Choosing to return home nearly a decade ago was a decision fraught with complexity and heartache. At that time, my career was ascending and on a forward track. Yet, the prospect of seeing my mother—a guiding light in my life—merely twice a year was a scenario I found utterly unbearable. The idea of her facing these struggles alone, with me so far removed from her daily life, tugged relentlessly at my heartstrings, compelling me to reassess what truly mattered.

Now, as I laid by her side, watching her struggle for each breath, I finally understood. I've become her caregiver, her advocate, her memory keeper. It's a role I've embraced with all the love and dedication I can muster. Each day, I fight for her, whether it's in the cold, impersonal hallways of hospitals or in the quiet of our living room, where I try to coax her into remembering, into being present, if only for a moment.

This journey has been marked by battles and victories, each one teaching me more about the nature of love and sacrifice. I've learned that love isn't just about the joyous moments shared in the sunlight; it's also about the quiet, often thankless tasks done in the shadow of illness. It's about staying steadfast when fatigue sets in, about offering comfort when fear clouds her eyes.

As the first rays of dawn filter through the window, casting a soft glow over the room, I reflect on the lessons this journey has taught me. Caregiving has shown me the fragility of life and the incredible resilience of the human spirit. It has stripped away the superficial layers of success and revealed my true essence—a son, first and foremost, deeply connected to this wonderful woman who brought me into this world.

With her hand in mine, as her breaths become more sporadic, I'm faced with the reality of her impending departure. The thought of a world without her warmth, her laughter, her unconditional love is almost too much to bear. Yet, amidst the heartache, there's a sense of peace in knowing that I've fulfilled my promise, that she would be leaving this world in her own home, in her own bed.

In the stillness of the morning, with her hand gently clasped in mine, I whisper a final "I love you," a son's tribute to his first and forever hero. It's in this moment that I truly grasp the measure of a life well-lived. It's not in the accolades or the public acclaim, but in the love shared, the lives touched, and the quiet moments of connection that define our humanity.

As I prepare to let her go, I realize that while we may lose the physical presence of those we love, their influence, their teachings, and their love continue to live within us, guiding us through the dark, shaping who we are, and offering comfort in the moments we need it most.

This, then, is not a story of loss, but a story of profound, enduring love—a testament to the unbreakable bond between a mother and her son, a bond that not even the final whisper of death can sever.

Return to My Roots

In the relentless buzz of WBNS's newsroom in Columbus, Ohio, amidst a fervor over a contentious governor's race I was reporting on, the insistent ring of my phone sliced through the day's usual chaos. On the other end was my sister Marianne, whose proximity to our mother made her the bearer of news from home. Her voice, a mix of worry and determination, abruptly shifted my focus from the whirlwind of political developments to our family's more silent struggle. 'Jim, when you get back to Arizona, keep an eye on Mom. Her memory isn't what it used to be, and driving… it might be time for her to stop.' Her words, delivered with care, struck me with a gravity I hadn't anticipated.

As 2014 waned, so too did the clarity of the path I'd been on. My career, challenging and successful, was up for renewal—a contract laden with promises and opportunities offered by a news director I both admired and respected. Yet, Marianne's call unearthed memories of a different time, a different place.

Back in 2005, the serene blues of Hilton Head and the leisurely pace of a weekend away had provided the backdrop for a conversation that now seemed prophetic. My dad, with a rare seriousness, had shared his concerns about Mom's future. "If anything ever happens to me, you'll probably be the one to take care of her," he'd said, the ocean breeze carrying his words away as quickly as they were spoken. I'd assured him without hesitation, not fully comprehending the weight of that promise.

Reflecting on it, his reasoning was clear. My siblings, all married with their own families and obligations, weren't in a position to come back home. Without my active participation, the decisions regarding Mom's care would likely involve relocating her or placing her in a care facility—options that would be deeply unsettling for her.

Now, with Dad gone and Mom's independence waning, those words from Hilton Head resounded with a clarity that was unmistakable. The decision before me was no longer just about contracts and career trajectories; it was about family, duty, and love.

The choice was made. I informed Channel 10 that I wouldn't be renewing my contract at the end of 2014. The decision was met with disbelief from colleagues at the TV station, and across the broadcast industry who couldn't fathom leaving a thriving career for uncertainties that lay in caregiving. But for me, it was a call to return to my roots, to the family home in Arizona that held the memories of a lifetime.

My broadcasting career, which had taken me across several states and into the homes of countless viewers, had come full circle, bringing me back to where it all began.

The transition was jarring. The rhythm of a newsroom, the adrenaline of deadlines, and the camaraderie of colleagues were replaced by the quietude of a home that now seemed both familiar and foreign. Mom's once sharp wit and vibrant stories were giving way to a fog of forgetfulness, her fierce independence shadowed by a growing vulnerability.

Mom's essence was defined by her caring and kind nature, a constant presence weaving through the very fabric of our lives with unwavering love and devotion. For all of my 57 years, she had been my closest friend, guiding me through every triumph and challenge, from the earliest days of grade school to the complexities of adulthood. Born in the heart of Van Wert, Ohio, in 1935, Mom's upbringing was steeped in simplicity and a deep-rooted love for family. In an era untouched by modern technology, she found solace in the comfort of books and the warmth of the kitchen, where she nurtured her culinary skills.

At just 15, Mom's life took a pivotal turn when she met my father, sparking a love that would stand the test of time. Their romance, rooted in the innocence of their teenage years, quickly blossomed, highlighted by moments like their first dance at the Junior Prom. It wasn't long before Mom, still in her youth, embraced both motherhood and marriage, tying the knot with Dad in her senior year. This marked the beginning of a shared adventure, filled with dreams and the laughter of four children—Mick, Bill, Marianne, and myself. In 1972, our family narrative took a bold leap as we traded the familiar surroundings of Ohio for the new horizons of Arizona, setting the stage for countless memories and the continuation of our family's legacy.

Mom embraced her artistic talents, using charcoal and pencil to beautifully depict the landscapes of juniper and pine trees in northern Arizona. Her interest in art extended to collecting Native American pieces, acquiring an array of vibrant paintings, intricately carved kachina dolls, delicate sand sculptures, and exquisite turquoise jewelry, all of which reflected the rich cultural heritage of the Southwest.

After relocating to the Colorado River area, Mom found new avenues to express her deep kindness by volunteering extensively with the hospital's auxiliary team. Known affectionately as one of the 'pink ladies,' she immersed herself wholeheartedly in her role, providing comfort and a friendly presence to those in treatment. She moved from room to room, not just offering a listening ear but also sharing her compassion, becoming a source of hope and light in the lives of many.

In her later years, Mom often conveyed to hospice workers how just a heartfelt conversation could lift spirits, prompting patients to shift from resting in bed to sitting up in chairs. This seemingly small action held profound significance, not only as a crucial step in their healing journey but also in enhancing their sense of self-worth.

In 1991, her selfless dedication was recognized on a larger stage when U.S. Senator Jon Kyl honored her with a Community Achievement Award for her "countless hours of volunteerism." True to her humble nature, Mom accepted the accolade with grace, dedicating it to the legion of deserving volunteers by saying, "there were so many ladies out there who were so deserving. So I accept this for all of you."

In January 2003, our family shared one of its most cherished memories when we gathered at Rex Ranch, just south of Tucson, to celebrate Mom and Dad's golden 50th wedding anniversary. This significant milestone unfolded over a weekend filled with laughter, enthralling stories, relaxation, and delicious meals prepared by an enigmatic Australian chef.

Over the years, Mom's nurturing spirit reached beyond her own children to embrace four grandchildren and six great-grandchildren, demonstrating her boundless capacity for love. Despite facing some challenges, Mom and Dad's strong bond endured, marked by an extraordinary 58 years of marriage until Dad's passing in 2011. After his departure, Mom faced the unfamiliar territory of solitude for the first time in her life.

For as long as I can remember, my mom was more than just a parent; she was my steadfast best friend. It seems almost surreal, but arguments between us were virtually non-existent. From those grade school days when we'd sit in my room with a cassette recorder, co-hosting our own music shows, to the times she organized lavish fundraising events at our home during my venture into politics—events attended by notable figures like Senator John McCain—she was always my rock

When I ventured into broadcasting at 30, her support remained steadfast. She would tune in to watch my newscasts online, eager to hold the Emmys I had won for reporting, which I immediately sent to her. Our bond was strengthened by deep conversations about life and dreams, peppered with our shared, snarky sense of humor.

The admiration for Mom extended well beyond just my own. During her grand 80th birthday celebration, Mick bestowed upon her the title of "the most wonderful woman in the world," celebrating her remarkable ability to withhold judgment. "It's rare," he noted, "to hear her speak ill of anyone—such a wonderful trait."

Bill, adding his own reflections, spotlighted Mom's elegance and her knack for punctuality, "She got us there on time and had a way of turning heads, getting whistles, even with just a simple drive around town." He fondly remembered, "Dad always knew he'd found a perfect life partner in her."

Marianne, reflecting on her aspirations, confessed, "When I was little, that's what I wanted to be when I grew up. I wanted to be my Mom." She proclaimed, "there just wasn't a better mother that I'm aware of."

Lynette, Bill's wife who melded into our family in the '70s, echoed these sentiments, noting, "Mom was always kind and generous, and you just loved her from the beginning." She warmly remembered how Mom "made you feel comfortable and welcome," calling her "the center of the family" and acknowledging that she was the magnet "why everybody gravitated back."

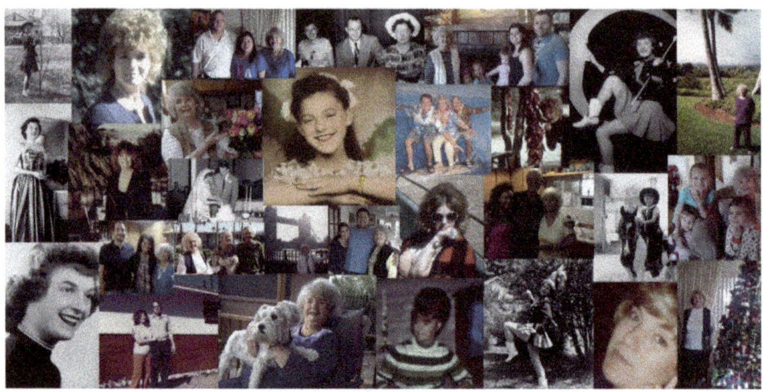

Each of these tributes, woven together, crafts a rich tapestry that celebrates Mom's enduring legacy.

Returning home to care for my mother, as she faced memory issues, was filled with uncertainty. Mom had always been a beacon of thoughtfulness, guiding me through life's challenges. But as dementia began to cloud her vibrant mind, a flood of fears overwhelmed me. The possibility of watching Mom lose herself to forgetfulness filled me with dread. I feared dementia would erase her memories, her laughter, and her spirit, leaving behind only a shadow of the woman I cherished.

Dementia is a cruel thief, slowly stripping away cognitive abilities and cherished memories. As a caregiver, I faced the heartbreak of potentially losing the shared moments and experiences that defined our relationship. What would happen to my soul if I became a stranger to her?

The progression of dementia brought not only emotional pain but also practical challenges—from managing daily care to navigating complex medical decisions. The unpredictable nature of the disease compounded the anxiety, leaving me to wonder if my mother would recognize me or retain any fragments of her past.

These fears haunted me, casting shadows over my hopes and testing my resolve. Yet, amidst this storm of doubt, one thing remained clear: the love between us was unbreakable. With this love as my anchor, I committed to facing the trials ahead, determined to honor and preserve my mother's legacy.

Reality of Family Caregiving

Deciding to come back home and look after my Mom has been an intensely personal odyssey, one that I've realized many other families are also embarking on. This collective journey is shaped by various elements, each threading through the tapestry of our lives in distinct ways.

At the heart of this trend is our aging society. With more of us living longer, thanks to medical miracles that turn once-fatal diseases into manageable conditions, the need for caregiving is expanding. It's not just about more candles on the birthday cake; it's about supporting a quality of life in those extra years.

Then there's the elephant in the room – the skyrocketing cost of healthcare. The price tag attached to professional caregiving facilities like nursing homes is climbing out of reach for many. This economic squeeze is nudging families toward a more heartfelt solution: caring for their loved ones at home.

There's something deeply comforting about being in familiar surroundings, especially in our golden years. Many seniors, my Mom included, cherish their independence and the memories embedded in the walls of their homes. This longing for home-based care calls family members to step into roles of caregivers, a task we embrace with love.

Technology, too, is lending a helping hand. Innovations like telemedicine and home monitoring systems are bridging the gap between professional medical support and home care, making the caregiving journey a tad easier to navigate.

Our changing societal landscape, with its bustling dual-income households and evolving family structures, is also reshaping caregiving dynamics. The traditional external support systems may not be as readily available, prompting families to lean on each other more heavily.

There's an undeniable personal touch to family caregiving. Tailoring care to the unique needs and preferences of our loved ones not only enhances their quality of life but also strengthens our bonds. It's about finding joy in the small moments, a shared laugh, or a quiet afternoon together.

And let's not overlook the deep-seated cultural and emotional currents that underscore caregiving. In many cultures, including mine, caring for aging parents is not just a responsibility but a profound expression of love and respect. It's a way of honoring the journey they've walked and the sacrifices they've made.

The path of caregiving, while a common journey for many, is painted with a unique palette of stories, challenges, and moments of grace for each of us. It's a deeply personal and meaningful role, shaped by individual experiences and motivations.

The conversation I had with my Dad that day back in Hilton Head left a deep impression on me, highlighting the emotional weight of potentially moving Mom into a long-term elderly facility against her wishes. Many of you might find yourselves facing this difficult decision due to your own family commitments, where integrating an aging parent into your household may not be feasible.

Let's be clear: There is nothing wrong with making such a choice, particularly if it's planned in advance. However, it's crucial to engage in these important discussions sooner rather than later. If you're in your 30s or older and haven't yet discussed future living arrangements with your parents, now is the time to set aside a moment and initiate this conversation.

Moving an elderly family member into a senior living facility can provide a range of benefits that enhance both their quality of life and the peace of mind for their families. These facilities offer professional care tailored to the specific needs of older adults, including medical supervision, assistance with daily activities, and medication management. Designed with safety and security in mind, senior living environments feature secure entrances, emergency response systems, and are staffed around the clock, crucial for seniors with mobility issues or those at risk of falls.

One of the significant advantages of these facilities is the reduction of household responsibilities. Residents are relieved from daily chores like cooking, cleaning, and maintenance, allowing them to focus more on enjoying their retirement. Furthermore, these communities foster social interactions through planned activities and events, helping seniors to combat loneliness and stay socially active.

Many facilities also offer fitness programs and recreational activities specifically tailored to seniors, helping them maintain physical health and mental sharpness. For those with specific health issues such as dementia or chronic illnesses, specialized care units are available with staff trained to manage these conditions effectively.

Additionally, the adaptability of senior facilities is a key benefit. As residents' needs change with age, the level of care can be adjusted, ranging from independent living to assisted living to full nursing care, all within the same community. This seamless transition in care levels ensures that seniors receive the appropriate support as their needs evolve.

For family members, the decision to move a loved one into a senior living facility can bring peace of mind, knowing that their relative is in a safe, caring, and engaging environment. This decision, while significant, helps ensure that the senior's later years are lived with dignity and comfort.

Again, it's better to have discussions about aging sooner rather than later, as aging is a universal experience that impacts everyone.

My personal journey to become my Mom's caregiver has been deeply influenced by my friend, Brad Dean. His act of donating a kidney to a stranger at a distant hospital profoundly moved me. This immense act of kindness showcased the power of human compassion, demonstrating how our choices can significantly impact others and shape our own lives. Brad's decision was driven by a profound sense of purpose and faith, inspired by the stories of individuals awaiting life-saving transplants. The effect of his generosity extended far beyond his expectations, greatly enriching the life of a 67-year-old woman and her family by extending her life for more than a decade.

Brad's humility and generosity are as remarkable as his quiet strength and inherent goodness, which have left a lasting impression on me, underscoring the extraordinary impact and rarity of genuinely selfless individuals in our lives and the immense impact of their actions on the world.

New Rules

My first act upon returning home was convincing Mom to relinquish her car keys. I braced myself for resistance, for the storm of protest that never came.

When Mom shared the story of her little misadventure, driving on the wrong side of those glaring orange cones placed by the local traffic crew, it was hard not to picture the scene. She recounted it with a sort of bewildered amusement, emphasizing how a "nice young man" had somehow managed to halt her wayward journey, gesturing emphatically for her to return to the right side of the road. Despite the gravity of the situation, I couldn't help but quip, "I'm not so sure he was just waving," trying to inject a bit of humor into what was clearly a distressing experience for her.

Yet, beneath the light-hearted exchange, a stark reality was setting in. The episodes where Mom would return from her solo drives to the beauty salon, her complexion pale and her hands trembling, were becoming more frequent. Each time she walked through the door, looking like a ghost of her former self, the weight of her vulnerability in those moments pressed heavily on my heart. It was becoming increasingly clear that these weren't just isolated incidents but alarming signs of her diminishing capacity to navigate the roads she once traversed with confidence.

The juxtaposition of Mom's casual recounting of her driving escapades against the visible toll they took on her painted a vivid picture of the growing challenges she faced. It was a transition that could have marked the beginning of a battle, a tangible symbol of independence lost. Yet, to my relief and surprise, Mom handed over her car keys with grace, an acceptance that spoke volumes of her trust and understanding of the situation. It was a moment I recognize as incredibly fortunate, a rare ease in the often-rocky path of caregiving. Mom, understanding the necessity, never voiced a complaint. In fact, she seemed relieved. This act marked the beginning of a new chapter, one where I became her chauffeur, her confidant, her chief assistant.

I understand now, more than ever, that this phase of caregiving—negotiating the delicate matter of when a loved one should stop driving—is a milestone fraught with emotion and potential conflict. It's a crossroads where safety intersects with autonomy, and the path chosen can deeply affect the relationship between caregiver and care recipient.

For those who might find themselves on the precipice of this challenging conversation, I offer this advice: approach the situation with empathy, patience, and clear communication. Understand that for your parent, driving is not just a mode of transportation but a symbol of independence, control, and identity. The prospect of giving up the keys can evoke a sense of loss, fear, and even grief.

It's crucial to initiate this conversation from a place of care and concern, emphasizing the importance of safety for both your loved one and others. Share specific observations that have led to your concern, and be prepared to listen to their feelings and fears about this transition. It may not be a single conversation but a series of discussions that gradually lead to a mutual understanding.

Exploring alternatives together can also ease the transition. I told my Mom I'd take her wherever she wanted or needed to go. Perhaps with your parent you could mention options like public transportation, rideshare services, or arranging for family and friends to help with transportation. The key is to acknowledge the loss of independence your loved one might feel.

For those facing resistance, consider involving a neutral third party, such as a doctor or a driving assessment professional, who can provide an objective evaluation of the safety risks. Sometimes, hearing the concerns from a healthcare professional can reinforce the message without the emotional charge it might carry coming from a family member.

Remember, every family's journey is unique, and what works for one might not work for another. Patience, empathy, and open communication are key. Know that you're not alone in navigating these waters, and that seeking support—from support groups, counseling, or caregiver resources—can provide not only strategies but also solace during these challenging times.

Our outings early on became the highlights of our days, from routine appointments to leisurely Sunday drives with the dog, each journey weaving new memories into the fabric of our lives. It was a semblance of normalcy in a life that was quietly shifting.

In addition to concerns about her driving, we encountered another troubling issue with my Mom. She had her computer set up downstairs and spent hours playing games like FreeCell and Mahjong. One day, as I was heading to the garage, I overheard her on the phone with someone discussing a supposed malfunction with her computer. The conversation immediately set off alarm bells for me, especially when the caller pressured her to reveal her credit card information to fix a computer that was, in fact, functioning perfectly.

I intervened swiftly, realizing it was a scam. I questioned the caller about the legitimacy of their company, but the vague and evasive responses only heightened my suspicions. This disturbing experience highlighted the urgent need for vigilance, particularly to protect elderly parents who may not fully understand the intricacies of modern technology. Scammers frequently target seniors, exploiting the stereotype that they have considerable savings, although even those with limited means are at risk.

The prevalence of internet and mail scams targeting seniors is indeed concerning. While one might hope that as more tech-savvy generations age, this problem might decrease, it's more likely that scammers will continue to refine their strategies to entice their targets, regardless of their familiarity with technology. Therefore, if you are caring for a loved one, it is critical to remain alert. Continuously watch for suspicious activities and educate your loved ones about the potential threats posed by online and mail fraud to safeguard them from these deceptive schemes.

To avert such situations in the future, we established a new rule: Mom would no longer answer calls from unfamiliar numbers. This precaution taught us to remain constantly on guard against potential scams, serving as an essential reminder for anyone responsible for the care of the elderly.

She is More than Mom

Stepping into the role of caregiver for my mother was a journey filled with lessons, some learned through laughter, others through tears. One of the first and perhaps most profound lessons I learned was to see my mother not just as a parent but as a whole person—a woman with desires, memories, and a longing for companionship that didn't fade with age.

I remember vividly one afternoon, as I was watching a football game on TV, Mom walked into the living room holding an old photograph. It was a picture of a gentleman, a friend of my dad's, someone from the tapestry of her past. She asked, almost tentatively, if I thought he might still be around, a question that, to me, seemed to come out of the blue. In that moment, caught off guard, I laughed it off, suggesting that he was probably long gone. Mom just nodded and retreated back to her room, the moment passing but not forgotten.

It wasn't until days later that the significance of that exchange truly sank in. That photograph wasn't just a piece of paper; it was a window into Mom's heart, a hint at the companionship she might have been yearning for. In that moment, she wasn't just my elderly mother; she was a woman reflecting on her life, pondering the possibilities that might still lie ahead. The realization hit me hard—I had missed an opportunity to connect with her, to acknowledge her needs and desires beyond the realm of health and care.

I approached Mom later, apologizing for my earlier insensitivity. We embarked on a small quest together, searching the internet for any trace of the man in the photograph. Though we discovered he had passed away, that search became more than just a hunt for a name; it was a shared journey, a reaffirmation of Mom's place in the world as an individual with her own set of desires and curiosities.

That experience taught me a crucial lesson, one that I feel compelled to share with other sons who find themselves in caregiving roles: Your mother, regardless of her age, remains a vibrant, living being with her own hopes, memories, and perhaps even a longing for companionship. It's easy to get caught up in the responsibilities and routines of caregiving, but it's vital to remember that our parents are more than just the roles they've played in our lives. They are individuals with rich inner lives, deserving of respect, recognition, and, when they express it, companionship.

From that day forward, I made a promise to myself and to my best friend—my mother—to never overlook her personhood. I vowed to nurture not only her health but also her spirit, encouraging her to pursue social engagements, friendships, and whatever else might bring joy and fulfillment to her days. This lesson, learned in the glow of a football game and the shadow of an old photograph, has stayed with me, a constant reminder of the depth and complexity of the caregiving journey.

Being back in the house where I grew up, surrounded by the echoes of a past life while navigating the realities of caregiving, was surreal. For years, at bedtime, I'd tell Mom 'I love you,' and she would quickly reply with 'I love you more.' In a playful bid to now have the last word, I began adding 'I love you more, 3,000 times.' A new twist to an exchange she never forgot. This intimate ritual, a stark contrast to the serious public persona I cultivated in my career, grounded me, reminding me of my roots and what truly mattered.

Finding the Finances

The early years back home were a time of adjustment, of finding a new balance. I turned to writing, channeling experiences and reflections into books that connected me with readers in a new, profound way. A YouTube channel became an outlet for creativity and connection, a bridge between my past profession and my present reality.

Dad's foresight in securing Mom's financial future with an IRA granted us a cushion that eased many worries, allowing me to focus on Mom without the looming stress of financial hardship. Yet, the absence of a clear future for myself, particularly concerning my own financial security, was a shadow that lingered, an unspoken question mark hanging over my decision making.

Navigating the financial hardships associated with caregiving for a loved one can be a daunting and emotionally taxing experience. For many families, the responsibility of caring for an aging parent or relative comes with significant financial burdens that can strain budgets and disrupt long-term financial plans.

One of the most difficult decisions families face is determining the best living arrangement for your loved one. Often, this involves weighing the options of moving the parent into your own home, moving in with your parent, or considering placement in a private or public institution such as a nursing home or assisted living facility.

Moving a parent into one's own home can provide a sense of security and comfort, allowing for closer supervision and more personalized care. However, it can also bring financial challenges, including the need for home modifications to accommodate the parent's mobility or medical needs, increased utility costs, and potential lost income if one family member needs to reduce work hours or leave the workforce entirely to provide care.

Moving in with a parent can alleviate some financial burdens, such as home adaptation costs and increased utility bills. However, it often comes with sacrifices to your personal space, freedom, and lifestyle. Over the nearly ten years I cared for my mother, I didn't take any vacations or travel far from home. In the beginning, we attended family gatherings together, but as Mom's condition required her to remain home, the thought of leaving her, even for a short time, became inconceivable. By my 50s, an active social life had become less of a priority than it once was, although this change might not resonate with everyone. It's crucial to recognize the potential personal sacrifices involved in making such a decision.

Opting for placement in a private or public institution may seem like a more straightforward solution, particularly if the parent requires round-the-clock medical care or supervision. However, the cost of long-term care facilities can be exorbitant, often exceeding the financial resources of many families. Moreover, public institutions may have lengthy waiting lists, leaving families with few options for immediate care.

In the face of these difficult decisions, families must carefully consider their loved one's medical and personal needs, their own financial resources and limitations, and the available support systems and resources in their community. Ultimately, the goal is to ensure the safety, well-being, and dignity of the aging parent while also preserving the financial stability and emotional health of the caregiving family members.

I must emphasize that managing the financial aspects of my mother's care would have been impossible without Medicare. This program played a crucial role in lessening the burden, taking care of expenses for hospital visits, home healthcare, and prescriptions. It truly was a lifeline. Seeing the benefits of Medicare firsthand— and I say this not as a political commentary, but as an observation on the wellbeing of our society as a whole—has made me wonder if our nation would benefit from extending such comprehensive healthcare coverage to all citizens. The challenges we face are not bound by political affiliations; the struggle of caring for a family member and the stress of financial uncertainty is an American issue that transcends party lines and merits national discussion.

Lake Havasu, a beautiful, remote part of Arizona, offered tranquility and a sense of community, but it also underscored a stark reality—my career in broadcasting, as I knew it, was a chapter closed. The possibilities of returning to that world dwindled with each passing year, the industry's relentless pace unforgiving to those who step away.

Yet, when faced with the decision to embrace caregiving fully, to commit to this path with all its uncertainties and sacrifices, the answer came easily. The warmth of Mom's smile, the twinkle in her blue eyes, and the kindness that had always defined her made any doubts evaporate. My role as her son, her caregiver, became the most important role I'd ever taken on—a role chosen with love, a definitive yes to a question that, deep down, needed no pondering.

Crossing Thresholds: The First Visit to the Neurologist

In the earlier years of caregiving, I found solace in decompressing from my broadcasting career and immersing myself in research and writing. Mom and I settled into a comforting routine, fairly independent from each other during the day but sharing dinners every evening and watching movies together. Those moments became my refuge amidst the challenges we faced. Sharing favorite movies and TV shows with Mom became a source of joy for both of us. Despite her memory fading, her genuine reactions made each viewing feel fresh and new, allowing me to relive the magic of those stories alongside her.

Monday evenings were brightened by the enjoyment of Mom's homemade dinners, and a cherished weekly ritual with Marianne and her husband Don. Before my return, Don had been helping out by taking the trash to the curb on Monday evenings—a task I gladly assumed. These gatherings quickly became more than just a welcome routine; they were often a highlight of the week, full of conversation and laughter.

However, as time unfolded, a subtle shift began to manifest in Mom's cooking. The once-flawless dishes started to miss a beat here and there, as though a key ingredient had been forgotten. During these moments, Marianne and I would exchange knowing looks, gently searching for tactful ways to explain our unfinished plates to Mom.

Gradually, and without any overt conversation that I can recall, the preparation of those elaborate dinners ceased. For a woman who had devoted her life to crafting countless meals for her family, with a collection of literally hundreds of cookbooks and recipes stashed throughout the house, this change was profound. While there was some discussion around relinquishing her car keys, the cessation of her cooking likely carried a silent, heavy emotional toll for her.

During that time, I ventured into writing 'Mylo the Panda,' my debut children's book, with Mom playing a pivotal role in shaping the main character. She was especially thrilled about our GoFundMe campaign and even suggested she star in the introductory video to demystify online donations for her peers. Our shared journey through various media forms, from the Super 8 reels of the '70s to the VHS tapes of the '80s and '90s, and eventually into the digital realm, always highlighted her innate ease in front of the camera.

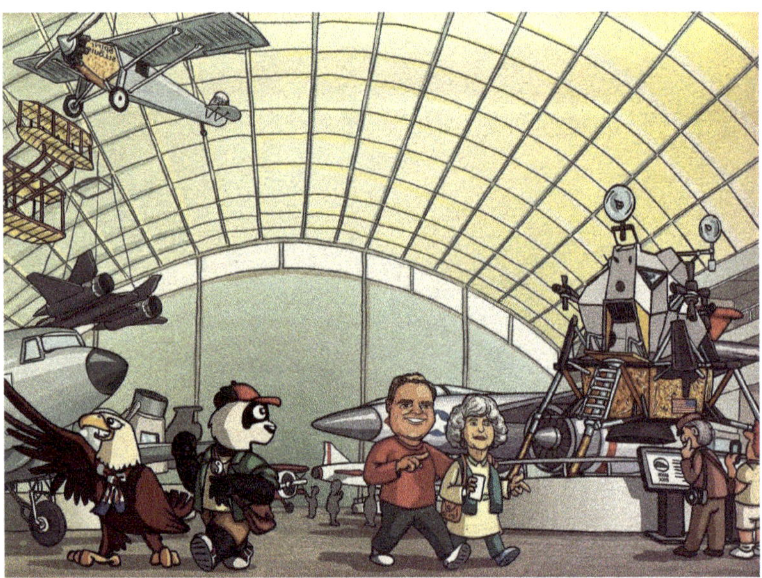

However, as we confronted the reality of her diminishing memory, we had to get creative. We simplified her lines, blending them with a musical backdrop to produce a video that was both heartfelt and polished. When she viewed the final edit, the joy and pride on her face were unforgettable, forever etching that moment into my memory. Her contribution added a genuine warmth and depth to our project, playing a crucial role in the overwhelming success of the Mylo campaign. One particularly poignant memory was her beaming smile after mastering a difficult line, despite the growing frustration she felt with the increasing number of takes required.

Mom was acutely aware of her memory issues. She often shared how, at times, she would lie awake in bed, disoriented and unsure of her surroundings. On occasions, I would find her standing pale-faced outside my bedroom door, far from her own room. I'd inquire, 'Mom, why are you here?' and she'd reply, expressing fear and confusion, 'I got scared in my room and didn't know where to go.' Witnessing the deterioration of Mom's memory was heart-wrenching, knowing she struggled, and feeling powerless to help. This significant change hinted that it was time to seek a professional evaluation of her memory.

The decision to take Mom to see a neurologist for the first time was fraught with a mixture of apprehension and hope. It marked the beginning of a journey, a step into the realm of medical assessments and diagnoses that we hoped would shed light on the subtle yet persistent changes we had been noticing in her.

The Mini-Mental State Exam (MMSE), a tool we would soon become intimately familiar with, was at the heart of this initial evaluation. Developed in the late 1970s by Dr. Marshal F. Folstein and his colleagues, the MMSE had become a cornerstone in the assessment of cognitive function. It was a 30-point questionnaire used extensively in clinical and research settings to screen for cognitive impairment and to estimate the severity of such impairment at a given point in time.

The test covered various areas including orientation to time and place, immediate recall, short-term memory, language use and comprehension, and basic motor skills. Each task was designed to probe different facets of cognitive function, making the MMSE a comprehensive overview of a person's mental state.

As we sat in the neurologist's office, the weight of the moment was palpable. Mom, ever the trooper, approached the test with a mix of seriousness and her inherent grace, despite the undercurrent of confusion that seemed to cloud her eyes more often these days.

When the results came in, Mom had scored a 19 out of 30. The neurologist explained that while this score did indicate some degree of cognitive impairment, it was not definitive on its own. However, it was a clear sign that we needed to pay closer attention and possibly prepare for a future where Mom might require more support and care. The reality was that mom's short term memory was rapidly deteriorating, but her older memories, most importantly not forgetting her children or earlier life, was intact.

This score, a stark number on a page, became a pivot around which our decision-making began to revolve. It was a tangible marker of the changes we had been sensing, an affirmation that our concerns were not unfounded. The score of 19 was in the low end of the mild cognitive impairment range, suggesting that while Mom was still capable of a degree of independence, the challenges she faced were likely to increase over time.

"At least you don't see a black wall," the neurologist quipped, gesturing towards the vibrant yellow wall that adorned the room. "When everything fades to black, that's when the alarms go off," she added, her tone a mix of levity and seriousness. Mom and I exchanged a glance, a silent communication passing between us—relief tinted with the gravity of her words.

The neurologist discussed the potential progression of cognitive decline, emphasizing the importance of regular monitoring and the consideration of lifestyle adjustments and support mechanisms to help Mom maintain her quality of life. We talked about cognitive therapies, social engagement, and the medication Donepezil was immediately prescribed to help stabilize her symptoms.

Donepezil is a medication commonly prescribed for individuals with Alzheimer's disease or other forms of dementia. It belongs to a class of drugs known as cholinesterase inhibitors. Donepezil works by increasing the levels of acetylcholine, a neurotransmitter in the brain that is important for memory, attention, and learning.

Subsequently, Memantine, another medication aimed at dementia, was incorporated into my mother's treatment regimen, though it appeared less impactful.

For Mom, Donepezil made a world of difference. It helped to alleviate some of the symptoms associated with dementia, especially her thinking and reasoning. By boosting the levels of acetylcholine, Donepezil improved her cognitive function and slowed down the progression of her cognitive decline.

It is important for me to note here that while Donepezil cannot reverse or cure dementia, it helped stabilize symptoms and improve Mom's overall quality of life. It kept her 'in the moment' while you were having conversations with her. Within a day or two of her not taking it, I would notice a huge difference in her mental focus.

As we left the office that day, I felt a heavy responsibility settle on my shoulders, accompanied by a deep resolve. The path forward was uncertain, filled with potential challenges and difficult decisions, but it was a path we would navigate together, armed with knowledge and a deeper understanding of Mom's needs.

Reflecting on it now, I understand that Mom had a clearer grasp of my caregiving role well before I did. She saw my dedication early on, even before I recognized its full extent. When we sat down and wrote her will in 2018, Mom suggested that the Havasu house should go to me alone because I was there to take care of her. I resisted this idea, insisting on including my brothers and sister, with whom I share a strong bond. I later found out they, too, had independently arrived at Mom's conclusion, but looking back, I realize I was in denial about the depth of my caregiving duties, secretly hoping for an 'escape hatch.'

The journey felt like piloting a plane with little experience, facing the inevitable need to land amidst unpredictable turbulence. For a while, I entertained the notion of a miraculous parachute escape, a way to avoid confronting the reality of our situation head-on.

Even now, after the meeting with a neurologist and faced with the reality of Mom's declining cognitive abilities, I couldn't imagine the magnitude of the commitment I had made. It was only in the second half of this decade of commitment that the full realization hit me – full-time caregiving is an incredibly stressful commitment, one that demands more than I ever anticipated.

As I stood on the brink of change, I embraced my role as Mom's caregiver with determination and love. Despite the challenges and uncertainties that lay ahead, I knew deep down that this was where I belonged – walking alongside Mom with complete dedication, no matter what the future held.

In the Shadow of Isolation: Navigating the Pandemic

As the world grappled with the onset of COVID-19 in early 2020, families everywhere were thrust into a reality marked by uncertainty, fear, and isolation. The pandemic's grip tightened, sparing none, but it was the elderly who bore the brunt of its cruelty, ensnared not only by the virus's lethal potential but also by the profound isolation imposed to safeguard their health.

For Mom, who had been navigating the turbulent waters of Alzheimer's with a semblance of grace, the pandemic introduced an unforeseen adversary. Prior to the world shutting down, she had been maintaining a steady, albeit fragile, hold on her memories and daily life, her cognitive abilities hovering around a score 19 out of 30 on the neurology tests—a concerning figure, yet not devoid of hope.

However, as COVID-19 unfurled its dark wings, bringing with it a veil of isolation that cut off vital social interactions, Mom's condition took a noticeable turn. Her short term memories quickly evaporated, while she began to struggle with the names of newer acquaintances and some longtime friends. Even our Monday night dinners with Marianne and Don were scrapped as everyone isolated, with the entire country literally shut down.

The COVID-19 pandemic hit our elderly community hard, not just because of the increased health risks posed by the virus, but also because of the profound social and psychological toll of the isolation measures meant to keep them safe. Seniors, especially those with existing health issues, were identified early on as particularly vulnerable, leading to strict isolation rules. However, according to health care experts, these necessary precautions came with unintended consequences:

Loneliness and Isolation: Lockdowns and distancing rules cut off seniors from their usual social circles, family visits, and community activities, leaving them feeling disconnected and alone.

Mental Health Struggles: The isolation and constant news about the pandemic heightened anxiety, stress, and depression among seniors, who worried about getting sick, accessing medical care, and what the future held.

Disrupted Healthcare: Routine medical services were disrupted, causing delays in treatment and management of chronic conditions as seniors feared going to appointments and risking exposure to the virus.

Cognitive Decline: For those with dementia or cognitive issues, the disruption of routines and reduced social interaction could accelerate cognitive decline and lead to confusion and agitation.

Physical Decline: Limited mobility and activity due to lockdowns and closures of recreational facilities led to a decline in physical health, worsening conditions like heart disease and obesity.

Digital Divide: While technology helped many stay connected, not all seniors had the skills or resources to use digital tools, leaving them more isolated than ever.

The pandemic highlighted, at least to us, the urgent need for better support systems to address the holistic needs of our elderly population during times of crisis, emphasizing the importance of social connection, mental health care, and access to healthcare services.

Christmas 2020 was particularly somber. The festive cheer that once permeated our home was replaced by a palpable sense of loss. The lack of physical presence of loved ones, the absence of laughter and shared stories around the dinner table, took a toll on Mom's spirit and, undoubtedly, on countless seniors experiencing the same enforced isolation. The stark realization that society's response to the pandemic, though necessary, had inadvertently cast a shadow on the mental well-being of the most vulnerable, was a bitter pill to swallow.

Amidst the chaos, Mom and I found solace in the small certainties we could cling to. We trusted in the science behind the vaccines, a flicker of hope in the overwhelming darkness. Yet, the silence of our quarantined existence echoed loudly, underscoring the profound impact of social isolation on mental health.

My mother and I always held a deep respect for science and the tireless efforts of health professionals. When the vaccines were rapidly developed and distributed as a bulwark against what seemed like a potential annihilation of the human race, we did not hesitate to support this scientific achievement by getting vaccinated.

However, it's crucial to address the other side of the coin—the profound isolation brought on by the pandemic, particularly for the elderly. This isolation, while necessary for physical health and safety, had its own detrimental effects, leading, in many cases, to lonely and heartbreaking passings.

I feel it's imperative to share these reflections in this chapter, not only as a testament to our experiences but also as a piece of advice for future generations who might face similar global crises. While isolation can be a crucial tool in controlling the spread of a virus, its impact on mental and emotional well-being, especially among the elderly, cannot be underestimated.

It's a stark reminder that in times of crisis, we must find balanced approaches that safeguard physical health without compromising the essential human need for connection. As we navigate these unprecedented times, let's remember the lessons learned and strive for solutions that preserve the integrity of our collective human spirit.

It was during these long, uncertain days that I came to terms with the permanence of my role as Mom's caregiver. The thought of stepping away, once a distant consideration, now seemed like an abandoned path, overgrown and forgotten. My life was here, in the quiet moments shared with Mom, in the routine of our days, in the silent battles we fought against the encroaching shadows of Alzheimer's and the invisible threat of a virus that had reshaped the world.

The initial ease of my decision to care for Mom, characterized by movie nights and casual drives, had evolved into a full-fledged commitment. I had become more than just a son or a companion; I was a caregiver, a protector, a constant in Mom's rapidly changing world.

As we navigated the uncharted waters of the pandemic, our journey was a microcosm of a larger narrative unfolding in homes across the globe, where families wrestled with the challenges of caring for elderly loved ones in the face of an unprecedented health crisis. The lessons were hard-earned, the losses profound, but amidst the trials, there was also a deepening of bonds, a reevaluation of priorities, and a renewed appreciation for the simple, unguarded moments of togetherness.

In the shadow of isolation, we found a resilience we didn't know we possessed, a testament to the enduring strength of the human spirit when faced with the unimaginable. For Mom and me, the pandemic was a stark reminder of the fragility of life and the preciousness of the time we have, a time we chose to fill with love, patience, and the quiet dignity of facing each day as it comes, together.

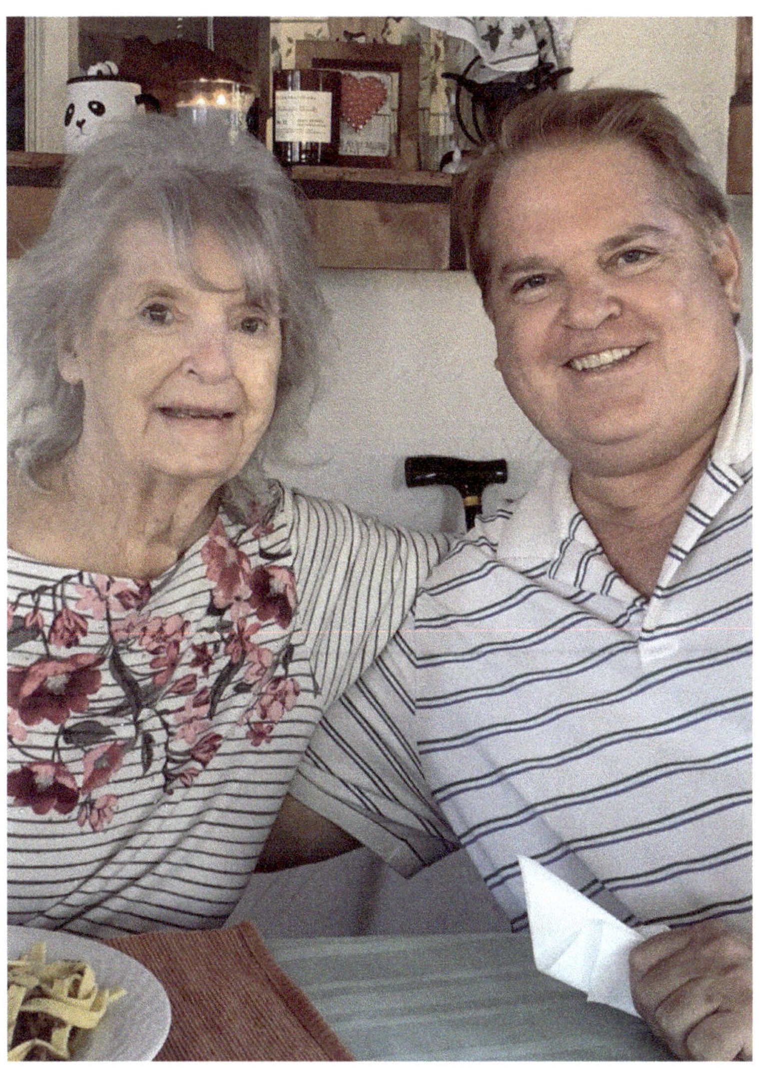

Shadows of Resilience: Navigating the Dark Terrain

As the world started moving again following the pandemic, the year 2021 for us unfolded as a dark and formidable chapter in my mother's health journey, marked by relentless battles with adversity and a series of harrowing trials. It commenced with a cascade of hospital visits that seemed to stretch endlessly, each one more taxing than the last. My mother, a beacon of resilience, bore the brunt of these tribulations, her spirit unwavering in the face of relentless challenges.

The insidious culprit that plagued her throughout the year was the dreaded urinary tract infection (UTI), a common yet often underestimated affliction among the elderly, particularly women. UTIs can stealthily infiltrate the body, wreaking havoc on one's health with debilitating symptoms. For my mother, a UTI spelled immediate weakness, mental fog, and a rapid descent into physical decline. Her once vibrant demeanor would be overshadowed by lethargy, her cognitive faculties clouded by confusion. The telltale odor in her urine served as a somber reminder of the relentless battle she faced.

Mom had earlier been diagnosed with stage 3 kidney disease. Her kidneys were moderately damaged and the inability to filter all the waste and fluid out of her blood resulted in ongoing high blood pressure. Everytime Mom went into the hospital for a UTI, her kidney failure level dropped to stage 4, forcing us to hold our breath and hope we would avoid kidney dialysis, which was one of her worst nightmares.

Throughout 2021, we endured the relentless onslaught of UTIs, each hospital trip leaving Mom weaker than before, her strength waning with each passing day. Yet amidst the turmoil of recurring infections, a far graver threat emerged – a diagnosis of rectal cancer.

Also known as colorectal cancer, Mom's rectal cancer had manifested as a series of malignant tumors in the tissues of the rectum, which is the final part of the large intestine. This type of cancer typically begins as small, noncancerous polyps on the inner lining of the rectum, which can eventually develop into cancerous growths over time if left untreated. Rectal cancer can cause various symptoms depending on the stage and location of the tumor, which for Mom included bloody stools, unintended weight loss, fatigue, and weakness.

The diagnosis of rectal cancer was confirmed through a series of diagnostic tests, including both a CT scan and MRI scan, and a tissue biopsy to examine the cells for signs of cancer. Treatment options for rectum cancer included surgery to remove the tumor and surrounding tissues, radiation therapy, chemotherapy, targeted therapy, and immunotherapy, depending on the stage and extent of the cancer.

Rectum cancer can be a challenging diagnosis for both patients and their families, as it often requires comprehensive treatment and ongoing management to control the disease and prevent its spread. The prognosis for rectum cancer can vary depending on factors such as the stage of the cancer, the individual's overall health, and the response to treatment. Early detection and prompt treatment are crucial for improving outcomes and increasing the likelihood of successful recovery.

This insidious disease, affecting countless individuals each year, posed a formidable challenge to Mom's already fragile state. A trip to Phoenix to consult with a noted cancer specialist left us reeling with disappointment as surgery was deemed too risky, sending us back to Lake Havasu with heavy hearts.

With chemotherapy ruled out due to Mom's compromised health, we placed our hopes on six weeks of radiation therapy to stall the cancer's advance. But even this course of treatment was fraught with setbacks, as yet another UTI reared its ugly head, forcing Mom back into the hospital and delaying her radiation sessions. Despite the radiologist's cautious optimism that Mom would probably enjoy "at least another year" the specter of uncertainty loomed large, casting a shadow over our hopes for her recovery.

As 2021 drew to a close, Mom completed her radiation treatment, rang the "cancer free" bell, her spirit undimmed by the trials she had endured. Yet, even in the throes of this triumph, another UTI struck (the sixth of the year), threatening to derail her progress once again. Frustrated by her medical team's reluctance to heed my concerns as Mom's primary caregiver, I found myself grappling with a sense of disillusionment. Why was my input not valued when I could clearly recognize the signs of a UTI after a year of grappling with them?

Mom's long-standing doctor, who had also been my physician during high school, parted ways with his medical team just before I returned home. Consequently, Mom was under the care of a family nurse practitioner for an extended period. This practitioner appeared disinterested in managing the comprehensive needs of her kidney, neurological, and cancer care. It felt as though we were lurching from one emergency to the next.

The toll of Mom's hospital visits extended far beyond the physical realm, permeating every facet of our lives with its relentless demands and unyielding pressure. Each time she was checked in, we found ourselves thrust into the disorienting world of hospital corridors and sterile rooms, where time seemed to stretch endlessly and the air hung heavy with uncertainty.

For four long days, each hospital admission—usually following a 9-1-1 call that brought an ambulance, fire truck, and police cars to our house—meant we would find ourselves in the cramped confines of a hospital room. The uncomfortable bed and chairs offered little relief from the relentless beeping of machines and the constant hum of activity just beyond the door.

Mom's voice, tinged with longing and confusion, would repeatedly express her wish to return home, her words echoing the stark reality we were all facing. Each time, Marianne and I would gently remind her of the necessity of her stay. The IV bags, dripping with antibiotics and hydration, were crucial for her recovery.

The relentless cycle of hospital visits took its toll, leaving us adrift in a sea of uncertainty and anxiety. In total, the time in the hospital and the emergency room amounted to over a month of 2021, our lives consumed by the sterile halls of the hospital, the constant barrage of medical interventions and tests a stark reminder of the fragility of life.

It was during this critical juncture that a hospital counselor intervened. With their guidance, I found myself in the office of a compassionate physician specializing in geriatrics, whose unwavering support breathed new life into Mom's care. Dr. Steven Massad's recognition of my role as Mom's primary caregiver empowered me to take the lead in managing her UTIs, providing much-needed relief from the relentless cycle of hospital visits.

A key piece of advice I would give any new family caregiver is to find an excellent Primary Care Physician (PCP). They act as the quarterback, coordinating all the healthcare aspects your loved one will encounter. Without a strong lead like this, managing the influx of medical information can become overwhelming. This is especially true for those without a medical background, as the complexity can lead to feelings of fear and hopelessness.

This newfound trust that Mom's new doctor placed in my judgment was transformative, effectively eliminating the need for any further hospital visits for UTIs during her lifetime. I became adept at spotting the early symptoms, swiftly administering antibiotics to tackle the infection head-on. This proactive approach allowed us to sidestep the emergency 9-1-1 calls and the frantic hospital dashes that, in the past, often came too late for an easy resolution.

To the medical community at large, I implore you to recognize and embrace the invaluable insights of family caregivers. We possess an intimate understanding of our loved ones' needs, rooted in a deep-seated bond forged through years of care and devotion. Trust in our judgment can pave the way for more effective and compassionate care, alleviating the burden on both patients and medical professionals alike.

The new partnership brought a wave of hope, yet the year had another twist when Mom and I got Covid before Thanksgiving, our first encounter with it. Mom's symptoms were mild, but mine were more severe, with a loss of smell and a lasting cough. It was a difficult close to a tough year.

As we embarked on the uncertain road ahead, I clung to the hope that the darkest days were behind us, and that the light of hope and healing would guide us forward. With each passing day, Mom's unwavering spirit served as a beacon of hope, illuminating the path.

Springtime of Hope

As the chill of winter gave way to the gentle warmth of spring, a renewed sense of hope blossomed in our lives, casting a radiant light upon the path ahead. The springtime of 2022 emerged as a beacon of promise, a stark contrast to the dark and tumultuous year that preceded it.

My mother, once ensnared in the grip of cancer unbeknownst to us, now stood as a testament to resilience and strength as she embarked on the journey of recovery. Her courageous battle against the unseen foe had left her weary but undeterred, her spirit buoyed by the promise of brighter days ahead.

Combined with a strategic approach to prevent the recurrence of UTIs, 2022 unfolded as a year of relative health and stability, defying the grim expectations that had shrouded its arrival. It was a year that seemed destined for loss, yet against all odds, it became a testament to the power of perseverance and hope.

With the progress in her treatments for cancer, dementia, and kidney issues, we even noticed an improvement in Mom's longstanding high blood pressure. Dr. Massad's effective strategies played a pivotal role in this positive shift, allowing us to move our attention from the more critical health challenges to the management of milder conditions, such as controlling her systolic blood pressure.

Although she was feeling better, the beginning of 2022 found my mother grappling with a profound sense of loneliness, exacerbated by the absence of her beloved schnauzer Bella, who had succumbed to illness in the midst of her own health struggles. The void left by her faithful companion weighed heavily upon her heart, casting a shadow over the holiday season and the dawn of the new year.

But amidst the darkness, a promise emerged—a promise of companionship and joy to come. We pledged to my mother that if she continued to improve in the spring, we would welcome a new schnauzer into our lives, a loyal furry friend to fill the void and bring light to her days once more.

As promised, as the flowers began to bloom and the world burst into vibrant shades of green and gold, we joyously welcomed a new member into our family—Ella, a spirited schnauzer who brought boundless laughter and love into our home. With a name reminiscent of Bella, chosen in a tender nod to Mom's memory (though she often referred to her as Bella, she graciously corrected herself when reminded), Ella quickly found her place in our hearts.

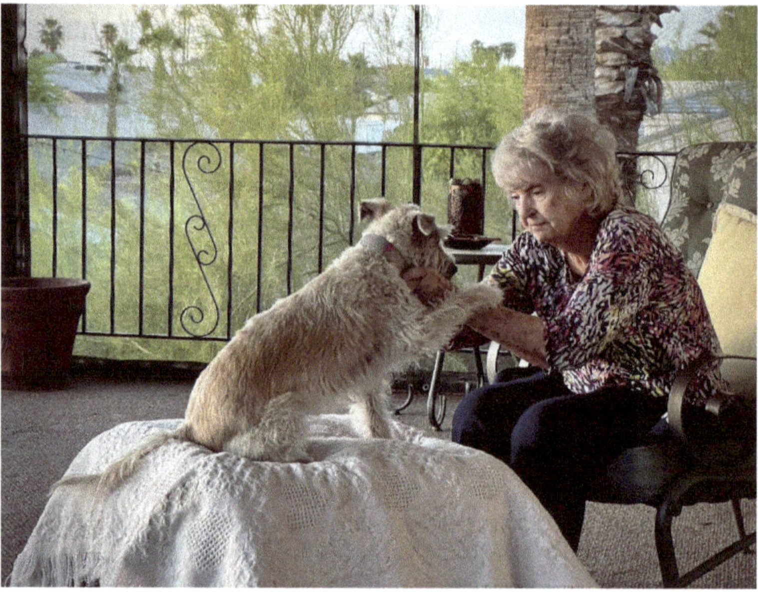

I've seen the profound impact dogs have on the elderly, particularly in my mother's life. Her dog brought immeasurable happiness and meaning, serving not just as a companion but as a steadfast partner. This companionship is invaluable for seniors, offering comfort, promoting physical well-being through activity, and instilling a sense of purpose and routine, especially important for those facing health challenges or isolation.

Dogs also provide emotional support that goes beyond words, understanding and responding to their owner's feelings, thus easing stress and anxiety. The responsibilities involved in caring for a dog, such as feeding and grooming, also offer seniors a fulfilling routine and a sense of accomplishment.

In essence, dogs are more than pets to the elderly; they're loyal friends who enhance their lives in countless ways, making them feel like cherished family members. My enthusiasm might hint at it, but I genuinely see dogs as earthly angels, silently enriching lives without asking for anything more than love in return.

Marianne and I embarked on a journey to California to fetch Ella from Coachella, which marked a turning point in my mother's journey, a tangible symbol of the hope and healing that had begun to take root within her heart. Despite the lingering challenges and the weight of physical limitations, she faced each day with courage and determination, her indomitable spirit shining bright.

Reflecting on that time, one of my most cherished memories is our daily ritual of sitting on the front porch, immersed in the unparalleled beauty of Arizona's sunsets. Each evening offered a canvas of vibrant colors, blending seamlessly into the horizon—these views inspired me to create a Sunset Calendar the following year, featuring amazing photographs taken from that very porch. As I watched, my attention would often turn to Mom. She sat quietly, observing the world unfold: cars rolling by, neighbors starting their evening routines, all bathed in the soft, radiant glow of the setting sun. Beside her, Ella lay contentedly at her feet. These peaceful moments deepened my appreciation for the decision to return home, enriching my connection with the simple yet profound joys of daily life.

Even though her strength hadn't fully returned, Mom embraced using a walker as her new way to explore the world. Each step she took, supported by the walker, was a small victory, a testament to her resilience and determination to keep moving forward, no matter the hurdles.

As she felt better, we joyfully brought back the Friday ritual that Mom so loved—her hair appointments followed by lunch with Marianne at a local restaurant. These excursions became the highlight of her week, offering more than just a change in scenery. They were opportunities for Mom to engage with friends and family, enjoy a fresh hairstyle, and indulge in a meal away from home. Though her appetite had declined, sharing a meal with Marianne became a cherished part of their time together, and to our delight, Mom would often surprise us by finishing her portion. Fridays soon emerged as the most awaited day for all of us, a weekly celebration of Mom's enduring spirit and the simple pleasures that brightened her days.

As the warmth of spring surrounded us, the shadows of the past year were replaced by the radiant glow of hope and possibility. The springtime, summer and fall of 2022 became a time of optimism, a testament to the resilience of the human spirit and the transformative power of love and companionship. And as we ventured forth into the unknown future, I held onto the belief that even in the face of adversity, there would always be moments of beauty and grace to guide us along the way.

Cut the Stigma

In our society, the role of caregiver has traditionally been painted with a distinctly feminine brush, often relegating the nurturing, caring, and tending to the sick or elderly to women. This deeply ingrained stereotype creates a significant stigma around men who step into caregiving roles, particularly when it comes to looking after an ailing parent. This stigma is not merely a superficial societal judgment; it is a generational legacy, woven into the fabric of cultural norms and expectations that dictate 'appropriate' roles based on gender.

Historically, sons have been seen more as the providers and protectors, roles that, while crucial, are distinctly separated from the intimate, daily care associated with the caregiver role. Daughters, on the other hand, have been expected to naturally assume this role, an expectation that overlooks the individual dynamics and strengths within each family. This dichotomy not only limits the potential for compassionate care but also undervalues the deep, nuanced relationships sons can have with their parents.

The stigma attached to men as caregivers is multifaceted. It stems from outdated notions of masculinity that equate emotional expression and nurturing with weakness. Men stepping into caregiving roles often face societal scrutiny, their masculinity unfairly questioned, and their efforts minimized or overlooked. This external pressure can internalize, leading many men to hesitate or even reject stepping into a caregiving role for fear of societal judgment or perceived failure to adhere to traditional gender roles.

However, as societal norms evolve, there is a growing recognition of the need to dismantle these stereotypes and embrace a more inclusive understanding of caregiving. Sons, just as much as daughters, are capable of providing compassionate, competent care. The bond between a son and a parent is no less significant, and the ability to nurture and care is not gender-exclusive.

A report presented by the National Alliance for Caregiving (NAC) and the AARP Public Policy Institute in 2020 showed that the majority of caregivers (67 percent) are still female, and "gender inequality remains a serious problem when it comes to caring for elderly parents."

Claiming a proper place next to daughters in the realm of caregiving requires a collective shift in perception, starting with challenging and changing the narrative around masculinity and caregiving. It involves recognizing and celebrating the emotional strength, compassion, and dedication that men bring to the caregiver role. Societal acknowledgment and support for male caregivers can empower more sons to step forward, embracing their role without the shadow of stigma.

As we move forward, it is essential for society to foster an environment where sons feel equally called and supported to care for their ailing parents. This shift not only benefits the individuals directly involved but enriches the fabric of our communities, promoting a culture of empathy, equality, and shared human experience. In breaking down these barriers, we pave the way for a future where caregiving is a shared responsibility, valued and honored regardless of gender, allowing families to navigate the challenges of illness and aging with unity and dignity.

For me, transitioning into the caregiver role for my mother was a natural progression of our relationship, eased significantly by the deep friendship we shared. This foundation of mutual respect, understanding, and genuine companionship made it not just a duty but an honor to step forward and care for her in her time of need. Our bond, built over years of shared experiences and memories, provided a strong basis for navigating the challenges that caregiving inevitably brought.

This experience has led me to believe that men who share a solid relationship with their parents are uniquely positioned to embrace the role of caregiver with grace and effectiveness. The depth of such relationships can ease the role reversal from being cared for to being the caregiver, making the transition smoother and more natural. It's about building on the existing bonds of love and friendship, transforming them into the bedrock upon which caregiving can stand.

I encourage other sons who find themselves in a similar position to mine to step forward and assume the caregiving role with confidence and commitment. The societal stigma that may have once made this choice seem unconventional or less masculine is rapidly eroding in the face of a more inclusive understanding of what it means to care for someone.

Being a caregiver is an extension of being a friend, a confidant, and a steadfast presence in your parent's life. It is a role that requires strength, yes, but also the kind of empathy, patience, and compassion that are born out of genuine relationships. For those of us fortunate enough to have such relationships with our parents, stepping into the role of caregiver is not just our duty; it's our privilege.

In doing so, we not only provide the practical support and care our parents need but also honor the depth and significance of our lifelong relationships with them. It's a testament to the enduring power of family bonds and a call to action for sons everywhere to embrace caregiving as a meaningful extension of the love and friendship they share with their parents.

From my perspective, the journey of caregiving has taught me invaluable lessons that I feel compelled to share with those of you who embark on this incredible journey of love with your parents. Firstly, I've learned that every family's caregiving experience is unique, and what works for one may not work for another. Patience, empathy, and open communication are vital in navigating the challenges we face.

Another important lesson is to recognize the individuality of our aging parents. Regardless of age, they remain vibrant beings with their own hopes, memories, and desires for companionship. It's essential to honor their autonomy and dignity, beyond their roles as our parents.

When making tough decisions about care, we must carefully consider our loved one's medical and personal needs, our financial resources, and the available support systems. Our goal should always be to ensure their safety, well-being, and dignity, while also taking care of our own emotional and financial health.

I've also come to appreciate the invaluable insights that family caregivers bring to the table. We possess intimate knowledge of our loved ones' needs and can offer unique perspectives that can enhance the quality of care they receive.

The late former First Lady Rosalynn Carter summed it up best: "There are only four kinds of people in the world: those who have been caregivers, those who are currently caregivers, those who will be caregivers, and those who will need caregivers." This perspective not only underscores the need for inclusivity across genders in caregiving roles but also stresses the shared responsibility society holds in aiding caregivers in their essential duties.

I want to wish all of the family members well who embark on this journey of caregiving with their parents. Breaking down gender barriers and fostering a culture of empathy and equity enriches our communities and allows us to navigate the challenges of illness and aging with unity and dignity.

Good luck to you. And remember, the doubts you will have about your decision making should always be replaced by the knowledge you made each decision with love.

'Luck' of Dementia

The unexpected relocation of Mom's neurologist to Las Vegas, along with her entire 'black wall' of expertise, sharply underscored the acute challenges of accessing specialized healthcare in rural areas. Suddenly, we were left with only one local neurologist, who had mixed reviews and a waiting list extending four months. This situation starkly highlighted the urgent need for enhanced healthcare resources and specialization in rural communities, ensuring that timely and comprehensive care is accessible to everyone, regardless of geography.

Amidst this dilemma, we were immensely relieved to find that Mom's primary physician had a background in geriatrics. This expertise became our saving grace, warding off potentially catastrophic repercussions for her mental health.

If you suspect that a loved one may be showing signs of dementia, it's crucial to take thoughtful and informed steps to address the situation. Observing and documenting any changes in behavior, memory lapses, confusion, difficulty in completing familiar tasks, and language problems can be vital for healthcare providers when diagnosing and recommending treatment. Gently suggest a visit to a healthcare provider for a comprehensive assessment.

An early diagnosis is crucial as it allows for the timely administration of medications that can slow the progression of dementia, potentially preserving cognitive function and quality of life for a longer period.

Educate yourself about dementia, including its symptoms, stages, and progression. Understanding what to expect can help you provide better care and make more informed decisions as the condition evolves. Encourage activities that promote independence and cognitive stimulation, adjusted to their current capabilities. Activities like puzzles, reading, and simple daily tasks can help slow the progression of symptoms.

Discussing future care preferences, legal, and financial planning early on is essential. Consider setting up a durable power of attorney and a living will—some of the first steps I took upon returning home. It's important to discuss long-term care options while your loved one is still able to participate in decision-making. Additionally, joining a support group can provide a network of advice, emotional support, and practical tips from people who understand what you're going through. These groups can be invaluable in navigating the complex emotions and logistics of caregiving.

As dementia progresses, it can affect physical coordination and increase the risk of falls or accidents at home. Making home safety modifications, such as installing grab bars in the bathroom and ensuring the home is free of hazards, can help maintain a safe environment.

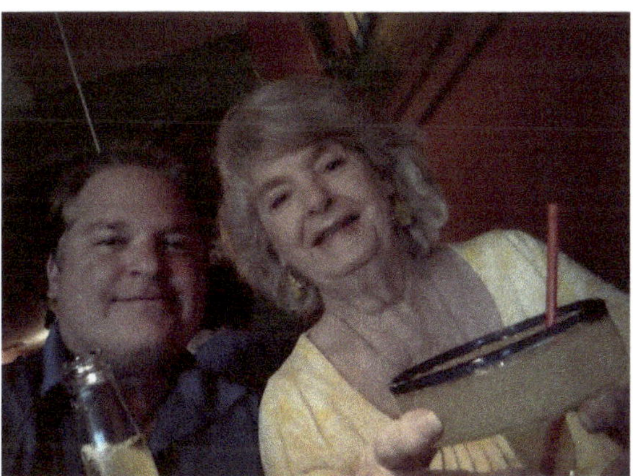

Our journey through the healthcare maze profoundly influenced our experience with Mom's disease, enabling us to discover rays of positivity amid the adversity. Her gentle decline stood out for its nature; unlike the more severe forms of dementia we'd witnessed in other close family and friends, her fundamental identity remained remarkably intact despite the advancement of her condition. This reality starkly contrasted with the grim forecasts we had been given, which spoke of that 'black wall' her earlier neurologist had mentioned.

The worst cases of the 'black wall' can manifest in a variety of deeply distressing ways. Individuals may no longer recognize their family or even themselves when looking in a mirror. They may lose the ability to communicate, and become agitated, confused and downright mean, posing a risk to both the person with dementia and their caregivers. Some wander off, while others are frightened by hallucinations. Additionally, the loss of basic motor skills can result in the inability to perform essential daily tasks, such as eating, dressing, and personal hygiene, leading to a complete dependence on someone else.

These symptoms don't just impact those struggling with dementia; they also impose a significant emotional and physical strain on their caregivers. Every day, I was haunted by the fear of the 'black wall'—how it could transform our relationship and, truly, whether I would have the strength to face it.

Mom's decline through the stages of dementia, marked by moments of lucidity and warmth, was a testament to her resilience and the enduring strength of her character. It taught us to treasure the fleeting moments of recognition and connection, each one a precious reminder of the person she remained throughout her battle with the condition. This experience also deepened our empathy and understanding for others navigating this difficult path and highlighted the unpredictable nature of dementia, where each individual's experience is as unique as they are.

Approximately 6 million Americans are living with Alzheimer's disease today, and according to the Alzheimer's Association, this number could escalate to nearly 13 million by 2050. Factors like increased rates of diabetes, obesity, and sedentary lifestyles can also contribute to higher dementia rates, as these conditions are linked to increased risk of cognitive decline.

Currently, there is no cure for dementia and no medication that can reverse its effects. However, there are treatments available that can slow the progression of the disease, **underscoring the importance of the earliest possible diagnosis.** This uncertainty can be daunting, as the path the disease will take remains largely unknown and out of our control.

Navigating the New Reality

As 2023 unfolded, the complexities of my mother's condition became increasingly formidable. Despite initially outliving the prognosis given by her radiologist post-radiation, our hopes dimmed as she faced fresh challenges. The relentless progression of dementia, possibly intertwined with a resurgence of her cancer, marked a steady decline in her vitality.

At this stage, hospice care became an invaluable source of support for us, transcending its often misconceived role as merely an end-of-life service. Instead, it offered profound comfort and assistance, signifying a pivotal shift in her care plan. We transitioned from pursuing aggressive treatments to adopting a palliative approach, prioritizing the alleviation of her discomfort and pain. Our primary goal shifted to ensuring her days were filled with as much serenity and comfort as we could provide.

It's worth noting that Medicare now reimburses certain patient navigation services in many states. These navigators are key in linking patients with their healthcare teams, coordinating care, and aiding with financial and legal matters. They also collaborate with insurers and key healthcare stakeholders. Local faith-based organizations might also offer comparable assistance, so exploring nearby options could provide you additional support.

For us, the hospice team surrounding Mom was a mosaic of healthcare talent—nurses, physical therapists, and memory specialists—who joined forces to tailor a care plan as unique as she was. Their collaborative effort was more than medical; it was a testament to treating the person, not just the illness, allowing Mom to face her journey with dignity and grace.

Pain management and symptom relief were at the heart of her care. The team wielded an arsenal of medications, therapies, and gentle, encouraging exercises to ease her discomfort. Physical therapy sessions, in particular, became islands of vitality in her days, often leaving her invigorated and able to enjoy a leisurely stroll around the house.

The journey through palliative care facilitated open, compassionate dialogues with nurses such as Kaisu Fisken, who uplifted our spirits and gently guided us towards understanding the forthcoming realities. In collaboration with Kaisu, Dr. Massad, and the entire caregiving team, we explored treatment choices, care objectives, and sensitive end-of-life decisions, prioritizing my mother's wishes at every step.

Seamless coordination across the healthcare spectrum ensured that Mom's care journey was smooth, regardless of the setting. The inclusion of memory specialist sessions, which Mom looked forward to, was a highlight, weaving joy and engagement into the fabric of her care.

One particular specialist, Jessica Stello, a Speech-Language Pathologist (SLP), made a significant impact on my mother's life. Through engaging conversations and memory challenges, Jessica not only stimulated my mother's mind but also provided her with a sense of purpose and connection to her own life journey. Despite her dementia rendering her short-term memory almost non-existent, my mother still retained the ability to make choices and engage in discussions, a testament to her resilience and determination.

Around this time, I gave a notebook to Mom and asked her to start writing notes to herself, aiming to keep her mind as active as possible. After it sat on the table for a week, I looked inside and found only one entry in her distinct handwriting:

<u>"Nov 2</u>   <u>Cloudy warm day</u>

I am sitting out on the porch. I don't have the slightest idea what day or time it is. It is a cloudy day but not cold. I have lost memory for the most part. It is a cloudy day with cool temp. Have a sweater on. Just hope the sun comes out soon. It's getting hard to write. Getting old happens but, one doesn't have to like it.

It's a cloudy cool day. Always makes me feel sad. Hope the sun comes out. I am so lucky to have this porch. I can see the lake and water and the cars go by. Also so lucky to have son Jim here with me. Also having a dog helps.

I just realized I have repeated myself several times."

The journal entry resonated with me deeply, particularly Mom's remarkable self-awareness in acknowledging her repetitions. Despite grappling with memory loss, she remained present in the moment, cognizant of her own fallibility. However, this realization also evoked a sense of sadness within me, serving as a poignant reminder that we were approaching the end of an era—Mom's tradition of meticulously writing birthday and Christmas cards, a cherished practice spanning decades, was gradually slipping away.

Jessica began administering the SLUMS test to Mom about once a month. The SLUMS test, also known as the Saint Louis University Mental Status Examination, is a screening tool utilized to evaluate cognitive function. It comprises eleven questions that assess various aspects of cognition, including orientation, memory, attention, and executive function, along with a brief evaluation of language and visual-spatial skills.

The conclusion of the test includes information about a couple named Jack and Jill, followed by a series of questions about them. Despite Jessica's efforts, my mother would never remember anything about the details she had just heard. Nevertheless, I couldn't help but chuckle to myself, knowing that even on her best memory days, Mom probably wouldn't have paid much attention to such a mundane couple.

There were moments when Mom displayed astonishing memory retention. For instance, when I asked her about a blue porcelain set scattered around various rooms in the house, she immediately recalled winning it in a raffle. The information she shared with hospice workers about her hospital volunteer days remained vivid in her mind. She never forgot her birthday, wedding anniversary, or street address. Moreover, she cherished the music of Dutch violinist and conductor André Rieu, often astonishing me by remembering all the words to songs performed by him and his orchestra.

However, her cognitive decline was evident. Her score on the MMSE test plummeted to single digits, and she struggled to recall her children's birth dates. She also forgot about an infamous hot air balloon crash she had experienced in 1980. Additionally, she seemed unaware of winning a trip to Hawaii, and even numerous summer vacations to Lake Powell with her family became a blur. Furthermore, she had difficulty remembering her grandchildren's names, while her great-grandchildren were completely lost in her mind.

By the beginning of fall in 2023, my mother's condition had deteriorated significantly. She was rapidly losing weight, and her strength had declined to the point where even moving from her bedroom to the living room became a monumental task. It was heartbreaking to realize that leaving home for her weekly hair appointments was no longer feasible. For as long as I can remember, those visits were a sacred ritual for her, a time to indulge in the latest hair trends, from the towering beehive to the elegant Jackie Kennedy bob, and even the lively curly afro of later years.

Navigating caregiving stress through all of this was a tough lesson for me. I knew about the positives of working out and eating right but often went for the easy options and skipped health checks due to insurance issues, leading to regular stomach pain which was, no doubt, stress induced. I did avoid alcohol and smoking and kept up my water intake, which helped. Staying hydrated is absolutely key. I learned to rest on tough days. My advice? Prioritize exercise and healthy eating. It's tough to put yourself first, but it's crucial for both you and your loved one.

As Mom's mobility decreased, she became increasingly housebound, and as her primary caregiver, so did I.

From Palliative to End-of-Life Care

As 2023 came to a close, the atmosphere of hospice care shifted. The transition from palliative care to end-of-life care signaled a profound change in focus and approach as my mother's condition advanced towards its final stages. While both stages aimed to provide comfort and support to those with life-limiting illnesses, their objectives and interventions differed significantly.

End-of-life care became the priority, focusing on ensuring that my mother experienced a peaceful and dignified transition in her final weeks. The primary goal was to spare her from unnecessary suffering or distress as she journeyed towards the end.

During this transition, the focus shifted towards managing symptoms and offering supportive interventions to maximize her comfort and quality of life. Practical aspects of care also evolved, with greater attention paid to assisting with daily activities and ensuring her physical surroundings contributed to her comfort and serenity.

Additionally, a support team came to my aid, offering a steadying presence through the increasingly complex emotional landscape. The stress, subtly and silently, began to manifest in physical ways that I hadn't noticed. A friend, who once praised my ability to look younger than my years during my broadcasting career, remarked upon seeing the changes in my physique and the thinning gray hair, "You finally look your age."

This transition to end-of-life care symbolized a collective effort between healthcare providers, our family, and my mother herself to ensure her final days were filled with dignity, comfort, and closure.

This moment was tinged with a deep sadness as it marked the end of my mom's journey with Dr. Massad. Her care was handed over to a hospice doctor, someone unknown to us, severing a bond we had come to rely on. As our primary care physician stepped back, we realized the exceptional talents of such professionals can sometimes go unnoticed. Dr. Massad was pivotal in extending my mother's quality of life and in understanding the pivotal role of her primary caregiver. Our appreciation for his empathetic care and support is beyond measure.

During this time, a crucial decision regarding my mother's medication arose. Her hospice nurse suggested discontinuing all of her medications, including blood pressure, kidney, and both dementia pills, which I was fine with initially, but when I briefly halted her Donepezil, her cognitive function rapidly declined. As her son and caregiver, I chose to keep her on Donepezil for the rest of her life. This medication helped her remain alert and engaged, enabling her to participate in conversations and stay present in the moment. To his credit, the hospice physician renewed the prescription without delay.

Anticipating every possible need, I developed a thorough plan titled "London Bridge Has Fallen," referencing the iconic landmark from our hometown, for my family to use following Mom's passing. This guide meticulously outlined the steps to be taken immediately, as well as a week, a month, and even further into the future. My intention was to equip Mick, Bill, Marianne, and myself with a clear, comprehensive roadmap to navigate through our grief, ensuring no crucial task was overlooked. I strongly advocate for such preparation.

In the wake of losing a loved one, especially after a prolonged caregiving period, it's common to experience a state of shock, where functioning normally becomes an immense struggle, regardless of how much one has prepared. Having a well-defined plan in place can serve as a stabilizing reference point during these overwhelmingly disorienting times.

Despite the trials of 2023, my mother never lost her innate kindness or grace. Even in the face of dementia and cancer, she held onto hope for recovery. In her heart, she wasn't ready to depart yet and was determined to take her final breath on her own terms.

Hospice care extended beyond physical support; it encompassed spiritual guidance as well. They arranged for a religious figure to visit our home, aiming to bring my Mom a sense of spiritual solace. This became particularly important after we shared a heart-to-heart conversation about life's profound mysteries, as she lay bedridden. "Do you think there's something beyond this life?" I asked, the weight of the question hanging heavily in the air between us. After a thoughtful pause, she responded with a simple "No." I echoed her sentiment, but we couldn't help entertaining a hopeful thought: "Wouldn't it be wonderful if we were both mistaken?" In that moment, we shared a deep reflection, intertwined with the bittersweet hope of someday reuniting with our departed loved ones, including my dad.

The visit from the hospice chaplain was something we both approached with open minds, perhaps as a chance for my mom to engage in a meaningful dialogue about faith. However, the conversation took a turn towards the oversimplified, almost as if the chaplain had preconceived notions about my mom's capacity for such discussions due to her condition. A fleeting glance from Mom, a silent communication in the midst of this one-dimensional religious talk, reaffirmed to me that this approach was falling short. It underscored that despite the decades-long presence of a Jesus portrait over my parents' bed, simplistic spiritual narratives weren't what my mom needed or wanted in those moments.

This experience highlighted the delicate balance in providing spiritual care that truly resonates with the individual's beliefs and experiences. It was a poignant reminder that the essence of a person, their capacity for complex thought and emotion, doesn't simply fade away with their physical abilities. In those final days, our spiritual reflections remained deeply personal, untethered from dogmatic simplifications, and anchored instead in the shared human experience of pondering the great unknown.

Faith can play a pivotal role in providing comfort, solace, and strength to families navigating the profound challenges of end-of-life care. Whether anchored in religious beliefs or a more personalized spirituality, faith can offer a framework for understanding, coping with, and finding meaning in the journey toward life's end.

Faith communities often serve as a vital support system, offering both practical aid and emotional solace, along with a sense of belonging. This support becomes crucial for families navigating the lonely journey of a loved one's decline.

My sister's story profoundly underscores this reality. As she grappled with the devastating journey of her husband's fight against brain cancer, the support from her Mormon church community became a cornerstone of strength. In the wake of his passing, they enveloped her and my young nephew in a circle of care and comfort, shining as a pillar of hope, particularly as she navigated this difficult period far from our parents.

In such trying times, faith transcends mere belief; it becomes a sanctuary for personal contemplation and prayer, bolstering resilience and providing clarity amidst turmoil. Moreover, it brings a sense of inner peace to family members, offering essential, albeit fleeting, respites within the rigorous demands of caregiving.

It's important to recognize that the role of faith in end-of-life care is deeply personal and varies greatly among individuals and families. Respecting each person's spiritual journey and beliefs is crucial in providing compassionate and holistic care at the end of life. For many families, faith can be a beacon of

hope and a source of comfort as they navigate the complexities of saying goodbye to a loved one.

As we approached the end of 2023, I reflected on the journey we had traveled together. It was a year marked by decline, but also by unwavering commitment and love. And as hospice shifted its focus, I braced myself for the inevitable, knowing that whatever lay ahead, my mother would face it with the same courage and grace that defined her life.

The Final New Year

A year had elapsed since Mom underwent radiation for rectal cancer, yet the signs that began to surface—blood in her stools, ongoing weight loss, and escalating fatigue—were pointing towards the harsh reality we had dreaded. By the winter of 2023, her vitality had waned considerably, transforming even the brief trek from her bedroom to the living room into a formidable challenge. We adapted our home to meet her growing needs, including the introduction of a wheelchair to aid her movement indoors. Over time, however, her strength to transition in and out of the wheelchair faded, necessitating our assistance. Each time we helped her, a groan would escape her lips, a testament to her enduring pain, even as she endeavored to mask it.

My mother's tolerance for pain was nothing short of extraordinary, akin to that of a superhero. She was the sole person I knew who could stroll into a dentist's office, undergo procedures like getting a bridge or crown, and never utter a word of complaint about pain. This stoicism extended to her hospital visits as well; she was never one to voice her discomforts. Thus, when the rare moments arrived where she'd grimace or release a faint sigh, it was a clear signal to us all of the immense pain she was enduring.

Also remarkably, as I have noted before but feel so grateful that I need to repeat it, Mom maintained her essence, her kindness, and grace, throughout her battle with dementia. Mom seemed to accept her condition with a certain peace, never succumbing to despair or losing her sense of self. This resilience, this refusal to let the disease define her, was perhaps the greatest gift she could have given me in those final days.

In the early days of December, I laid out a variety of photographs for Mom to select for her annual Christmas card. The options included happy images with her dog and vibrant flowers. However, there was one distinct photo that stood out: it captured Mom from behind, standing by the Christmas tree with her cane, looking out the door at a stunning sunset. When she singled out this photo for her card, I hesitated and asked for confirmation. With a gentle, yet somber nod, she affirmed her choice. It felt as if she was imparting a silent farewell through this image, sending wishes for joyful Christmases to our loved ones in the times ahead, despite her own absence.

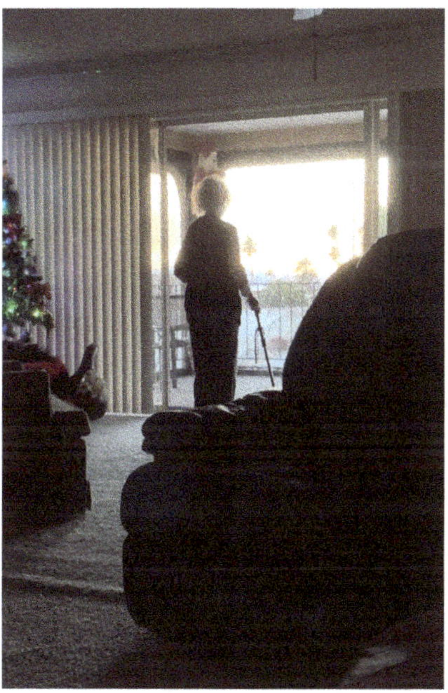

One final time I decorated our home with every festive ornament Mom had amassed over the years, and the collection was vast. Holiday cheer touched every nook and cranny. I even repurposed old curtain hooks from the living room to display extra Christmas tree ornaments.

Our evenings evolved into cherished rituals, where I'd guide Mom's wheelchair through the house. She'd take in the familiar decorations, each piece a fragment of the happiness and warmth they'd brought to our family over the years.

After spending months compiling and editing all our family's holiday footage—from Super 8 films of the '60s & '70s to VHS tapes of the '80s and '90s, and more contemporary digital recordings—each evening we'd immerse ourselves in those happy memories, with Mom delighting in the sights of her family's togetherness during what was her favorite time of year.

In a special moment in mid-December, I managed to record Mom one last time as she conveyed heartfelt Christmas greetings to her Facebook friends, complete with a Santa hat for added festivity. After reviewing the edited video, she voiced concern that she hadn't smiled enough, her unwavering perfectionism still shining through.

In the wake of the New Year, a faint glimmer of our old life shone through as Mom managed to join the entire family in the living room for Christmas dinner, and once again for New Year's Eve. We rearranged our space, bringing the dining to her comfort zone by the couch, since sitting at the table had become too uncomfortable. Mom always cherished family gatherings, reveling in the laughter, conversations, and hearty dinners.

Several years earlier, Mom passed the kitchen torch to her grandson, Cody. With gusto and adeptness, he stepped up, dishing out heaping helpings of beef and noodles, a dish that had long held a special place at our family table. Alongside him, Marianne dedicated herself to crafting our signature family dessert: a sumptuous chocolate cake with caramel frosting, meticulously following Mom's beloved recipe down to the last detail.

However, this year, as the noise of the holidays swirled around her, Mom mostly retreated into playing games on her tablet, eager to participate in the festivities but grappling with extreme weakness and the challenge of recognizing family members and friends who were no longer as quickly familiar.

After their Christmas visit, my niece Mallory and her boyfriend Will came to say goodbye to Mom, who was resting in her bedroom. "Well, you're pretty brave to be here," Mom quipped to Will. When he looked puzzled, she gestured towards herself and said, "you know, all this." Having always been meticulous in her appearance, her remark highlighted her enduring sharp wit and a touch of sad resignation, reflecting her acceptance of the changes she faced.

A photograph taken on New Year's Eve, showing her surrounded by family, would sadly be the last one of her out of bed. By the first week of January 2024, Mom was bedridden, solemnly marking the beginning of full-time hospice care.

Preparing for Goodbye

Initially, under Medicare's plan, Mom was granted hospice support three times a week, which soon escalated to daily nurse visits, further bolstered by independent home care assistance twice a day. With each passing day, the imminent approach of the end became unmistakably evident. The lead hospice nurse, pragmatic in her approach, introduced a regimen of hydrocodone and morphine, urging their use. The transition to such potent medication was abrupt, more so than I found comfortable. I yearned for an approach more tailored to our unique situation, honoring the distinctive journey Mom and I shared, marked not by rush but by a deep reverence for each moment we had together.

Yet, amidst this, Mom's spirit flickered strong; she continued to indulge in her Mahjong games on her tablet, a testament to her alertness even in her diminished state. I found solace in watching her engage with the game, her victories on the beginner level serving as small, yet significant, triumphs.

I endeavored to create a sanctuary for her in her room, adorning it with elements that brought her joy. Her favorite things, flowers for a pop of color she could see from her bed, photographs of her family, canvas paintings of sunsets, candles and nice scents, and the comforting presence of her dog Ella by her side. Nightly, we maintained our ritual of watching a movie together, or André Rieu who she adored, a semblance of normalcy in the midst of our profound change.

With Mom confined to bed, our mornings were often filled with the dramatic proceedings of court shows like Judge Judy, People's Court, and our personal favorite, Hot Bench. We would watch them together, often enjoying peanut butter toast and a hot cup of coffee. These shows, brimming with heated exchanges and courtroom battles, somehow became our unlikely source of entertainment and, in a way, companionship.

One afternoon, perhaps influenced by the confrontational nature of these programs, I shared with Mom my growing irritation towards one of our neighbors. They had embarked on constructing a deck at the back of their house in November, and by the holiday season, our backyard view had devolved into a scene reminiscent of a neglected construction site, complete with scattered debris and unfinished structures. I told her I was composing an angry text to let them know what an awful situation they had created.

Mom listened as I vented, her calm demeanor a stark contrast to my frustration. With a gentle voice she offered her perspective. "Send them a message" she suggested, "but frame it as a question. They might not realize the extent of the mess left by the construction crew. Ask them if they're aware, without laying blame." Her advice, steeped in a lifetime of navigating disputes with grace, immediately made me smile. I took a deep breath, composed the text, and followed her lead.

The response from our neighbors was unexpectedly warm and apologetic, far more so than I had envisioned. In the course of our exchange, I uncovered a poignant connection—like Mom, a member of their household was engaged in a battle with cancer. Had I given in to my initial instincts, I would have only exacerbated the situation, ending up with deep-seated regret.

Even in her fragile state, Mom continued to be a beacon of humanity and compassion. Her steadfast belief in 'kindness first' not only averted a needless conflict but also reinforced the transformative power of empathy and understanding. The world, indeed, would be a far greater place under the guidance of the gentle wisdom and patience exemplified by souls like my mother.

With her memory increasingly unreliable, Mom sometimes forgot her own fragility. One evening, I entered her room and found her standing by her bed, wracked by a severe seizure. The fear of her having a stroke—a worry that had haunted me persistently—immediately terrified me. I rushed to her aid, trying to guide her gently back to bed, but as she began to falter, my strength seemed insufficient against her unexpected weight. She collapsed, her body still shaking, eyes rolled back into her head, compelling me to frantically call 9-1-1 in a state of sheer panic.

The operator's calm voice cut through my fear, helping me back to a semblance of calm as I awaited the emergency team's arrival. Their professionalism and reassurance were a godsend in those chaotic moments, gently lifting Mom back into her bed. A paramedic reassured me on the side, affirming that her vital signs were stable, which comforted me enough to continue with hospice care rather than rush her to the hospital. After the chaos, Mom, utterly exhausted, fell into a deep, restful sleep and didn't remember any of it when she woke up in the morning.

The incident left me determined to prevent a recurrence. The next day, I installed a security camera in her room, a watchful eye to monitor her movements and ensure her safety. It seemed Mom understood this precaution too, for she never again tried to leave her bed on her own. This initiated a new habit for me: vigilantly watching the camera feed any time I was away from her side.

As the days trickled into mid-January, Mom's resolve began to wane; she ate her last piece of peanut butter toast and ceased eating altogether. Her fondness for blue cherry Gatorade, and its sugar and electrolytes, would keep her alive for weeks, astounding every nurse who visited her. The decision to stop eating, I believe, was her dignified response to the indignities of her condition. It was a silent refusal, born out of a desire to maintain whatever control she had left over her life.

The home health care workers had been responsible for changing Mom's diaper twice a day once she became bedridden. However, there were moments when I noticed she had urinated, her ability to control her bladder slipping away. Despite my previous reluctance to consider ever changing or cleaning my mom, the psychologically uncomfortable issue suddenly became irrelevant. With my best friend nearing the end of her life, I couldn't bear the thought of Mom lying in her own urine. Thus, there were times when I took it upon myself to change her, albeit not as efficiently as the professionals, but with the same love and care that Mom had shown me when I was in diapers. It was a profound realization of the circle of life, where we weren't ashamed but rather focused on ensuring Mom's physical well-being with the utmost dignity possible.

As time grew scarce and Mom's capacity to communicate diminished, she received phone messages from longtime friends. Yet conversations had become a struggle, her weakened throat muscles reducing her voice to a whisper. Communicating that her life was nearing its end was a difficult and delicate task. When we sent out that emotional Christmas card to family and friends, featuring her silhouette against a December sunset, we hoped the message was implicitly clear: time was running out.

One of the most heartrending moments in those final weeks was facilitating the last conversation between Mom and her 95-year-old brother, Dillon. Despite the physical distance and past disagreements, which they had overcome—reconciling with tears during a poignant reunion in Columbus in 2009—their final exchange was deeply moving.

I greeted my uncle, then informed him that Mom was listening. He reminisced about memories they had shared, and expressed the sorrow he felt from his wife's recent passing, a revelation that brought a tear to Mom's cheek. As the conversation wound down, their exchange of "I love yous" was tender and heartfelt. After hanging up, Mom's glance conveyed the heavy realization that this was their final farewell. Though she might have wished for greater closeness, their journey together was long and interwoven with the legacy of their loving parents.

Day after day confined to her bed, Mom started to lose sensation in her legs. We tried different pillows each day to elevate them, hoping to stimulate blood flow. There were moments she felt almost paralyzed, prompting me to massage her legs, feet, and toes—sometimes with considerable pressure—until she regained a slight sense of feeling. Any movement caused her discomfort. When positioning a pillow under her, I'd ask her to embrace me tightly so I could shift her in one smooth motion, yet she'd hesitate, worried it might cause me pain instead. Even in her own time of need, her concern was always for the wellbeing of others before her own.

Several months earlier, I introduced a white marker board in Mom's room that displayed the date and counted down to special events like holidays and birthdays. As Valentine's Day approached, I asked her if she would be my Valentine, quietly wondering if we would have that much time together. Her affirmation was weak, but she persevered and made it to the day. Since college, I had sent Mom flowers for special occasions, and since returning home, I made sure the house was always filled with them. This time, when I bought two dozen red roses for Valentine's Day, the weight of the moment hit me—the painful finality of the gesture was overwhelming. These roses would be the last I would ever buy for her, and the realization was emotionally devastating.

As I witnessed Mom's failing body and heard her fading voice, panic gripped my mind. The thought of calling 9-1-1 and rushing her to the hospital, hoping for a miraculous recovery, haunted my restless nights. I kept questioning myself, "Am I truly doing everything I can to keep her alive?"

For those confronting similar experiences with a loved one, understand that your fear is valid, and you are not alone. The weight of potentially making mistakes in these final moments was a constant concern. Additionally, there is the added pressure of recognizing that end-of-life caregiving is likely one of the most significant responsibilities you will ever undertake.

All caregivers, in their solitude and exhaustion, must prioritize their mental and physical well-being—a task easier said than done. Our fear of the unknown, compounded by a culture that often shies away from discussions about death, can be paralyzing. It's essential to acknowledge our limitations and seek help when needed.

In those moments when the dread of potentially losing Mom and the unknowns of what lay ahead seemed insurmountable, I found myself precariously close to the edge. It was then I recognized the profound importance of the supportive text messages from family and hugs shared with my sister and friends.

Each time I felt on the verge of losing control, I summoned my practical side for reassurance. I reminded myself of Mom's firm resolve to not end her battle with dementia, cancer, or kidney failure confined to a hospital bed, away from the comfort of our home and her cherished Ella. This decision to remain at home, made during clearer moments, was deeply anchored in maintaining her quality of life. 'Stick to the plan,' I would tell myself, striving to quell the rising tide of doubts.

There came a moment a week before her death, encouraged by hospice, for me to discuss with her that it was alright to let go, but it was a conversation she wasn't ready for. Her indomitable spirit shone through her frailty, as she watched me hold back tears, asserting that she wasn't going anywhere just yet. It was a moment of clarity, of defiance against the inevitable, that I couldn't help but respect. To the end my mom held out hope that she would get better. She never wanted to leave.

Yet, the decline was rapid from there. The final days were a delicate dance of presence and impending absence, of holding hands and shared whispers in the dim glow of her room. Her acknowledgment of her own mortality just days before her death was both heartbreaking and profound.

The cessation of her Gatorade intake marked the beginning of the end. Experts tell you the end of hydration starts the countdown clock for life at 72 hours or less. On that poignant day, I chose to recapture a piece of my youth, dyeing my hair back to the rich, dark brown of my earlier years. As the afternoon light waned, my mother stirred from her slumber. With eyes as blue and luminous as ever, she gazed at me—a tender mix of recognition and surprise. "My handsome son," she murmured softly, her voice weaving the warmth of a thousand memories into those three simple words.

Unbeknownst to me, those words would mark our final exchange, a cherished moment frozen in time, sealing our lifelong bond with her loving affirmation.

On the eve of her passing, I made a decision that I've since come to deeply regret—a decision born out of hope but shadowed by naivety. In the realm of caregiving, playing God is a grave mistake, a lesson I learned in the most heart-wrenching way. My father, during his final days in hospice care, had a moment of surprising lucidity before he passed, a moment I desperately wished to recreate with my mom. Thus, in those dwindling hours, I began to reduce the morphine doses I had been diligently administering, clinging to the hope of one last moment of connection, one final conversation.

The hours that followed were shrouded in a mix of anticipation and unease. At midnight, with the room softly illuminated by candlelight, Mom remained unresponsive beside me. By 3 am, a faint snoring filled the silence, a sound I initially found comforting but later understood to be the ominous 'death rattle,' a harbinger I had failed to recognize. My father had exhibited a similar sign, yet

Mom's was so subtle, so gentle, that its true significance eluded me.

At dawn, around 7:30 am, I was abruptly awakened by the sight of Mom struggling to breathe, her eyes open wide with what looked to me like an unspoken plea for help. Panic surged through me as I grasped the weight of the situation. I dashed to the refrigerator for the morphine, driven by a mix of urgency and despair. Later, a hospice nurse reassured me that Mom was not in pain and that such struggles were a natural part of dying. Despite this assurance, the image is etched in my memory, refusing to fade.

I share this deeply personal and painful experience to offer a window into the complexities and uncertainties that accompany the final moments of a loved one's life. If you've journeyed with me through this narrative, seeking understanding and solace in the face of impending loss, know that the path is fraught with challenges and choices that weigh heavily on the heart.

My hope is that by revealing this part of my story, I can provide some guidance, or at least solace, in acknowledging that in our most human moments, we are all searching for connection, for closure, and ultimately, for peace in the face of the inevitable.

The end arrived softly, moments after I gave her the final dose of morphine. My brother Mick, alongside his wife Johanna, joined us in Mom's room, bearing witness to her serene departure, as graceful as one could imagine. When her soft breaths faded into silence, we tenderly closed her eyes. Marianne arrived soon after, and together, we kept a quiet vigil beside Mom, embracing the belief that life's essence takes its time to fade.

Looking at my mother lying peaceful in her bed I realized my time with her had ended. Having navigated this flight for nearly a decade, unprepared at first, it had reached its destination and landed, meeting the goal my mother had envisioned all along: To

die on her own terms, surrounded by love, in her own house, in
her own bed.

Death is not the opposite of life, but a part of it. • Haruki Murakami

Moving Forward, Slowly

My mother's decades of community service in the town she'd called home since the 1970s were commemorated with a front-page article in the local paper, paying tribute to her remarkable contributions.

Six days after Mom's passing, Mick, Marianne, my niece Hayle, her husband Erik, and I bid our final farewells to her at a private cremation service, honoring her wishes. Witnessing her for the last time stirred a mix of beauty and profound sorrow. While I'm uncertain if I'd recommend this experience to others, it undeniably granted us a sense of closure. Someday in the future, as per her wishes, we will scatter her ashes alongside my father's, somewhere on land, as she used to joke, "just not anywhere near water"—an amusing nod to the fact that Mom never learned how to swim.

Weeks later, our family gathered for two celebrations in her honor—one public, one private—both of which she would have cherished. Despite feeling her absence intensely, there was a palpable sense of her spirit among us. The fact that every member of the family felt the need to come together in her memory stands as a testament to how deeply loved she was by each and every one of us.

Then, after everyone departed, a serene stillness settled.

The raw edges of my grief are palpable, with every corner of the house reminding me of her absence. The silence where her laughter once filled the air now feels like a void that grows with each passing day. I find myself missing even the challenges of caring for her, alongside the daily routines and the sense of protection I provided.

The process of mourning has unfolded gradually, marked by tears shed in the most unexpected places: amidst the aisles of a grocery store at the sight of an elderly mother with her son, at every sunset that reminds me of the countless ones we watched together, while gazing at a distinct painting of a Native American woman—a painting my mother always said would watch over me long after she was gone, and during fleeting moments of movies that have become difficult to watch without her presence.

Eventually, it came time to sort through her closets and drawers and decide what to do with her extensive collection of clothes and personal items. Thankfully, Marianne was there to help, and we took several days, spaced weeks apart, to handle this emotional task. We chose to donate many of Mom's belongings to the local Hospice store, hoping others might find use for them. As we moved on to her desk drawers, I discovered newspaper clippings of family members she had kept for decades, a testament to her immense pride in her family.

Ella, our faithful companion, also deeply feels the loss. She sits at the top of the stairs, expectantly waiting for Mom to return, a ritual that underscores the profound emptiness left behind. Sometimes, she simply sits and stares at me, as if telepathically asking what happened to the wonderful person she loyally guarded each night since we brought her home as a puppy from Coachella.

The ripple of grief extends beyond myself, touching every family member. Mick, Bill, Marianne, and I are united in our sorrow, as are Hayle, Cody, Mallory, and Billy, who mourn the absence of their grandmother. Her loss has created a gap that will never fully close, leaving us with only memories—memories that will become particularly vivid during the holidays, the joy of shared meals, the excitement of presents, and those memorable treks to Dillard's. Each memory is a reminder of her inherent kindness and warmth.

After stepping away from my broadcasting career to care for Mom, I've learned invaluable lessons about the strength found in the act of caregiving. These lessons have reshaped my understanding of life, emphasizing the importance of compassion and the deep connections forged through unconditional love.

As I reflect on these lessons, I'm compelled to share them, hoping they can light the way for others. The insights gained from this journey of love and loss may offer comfort and understanding to those navigating their paths toward a final goodbye.

Amidst this sorrow, an unexpected and peculiar incident occurred, providing a fleeting moment of comfort—a subtle, almost ethereal whisper from beyond, which I find myself grappling to fully understand.

I've never been one to delve into spiritual realms or entertain mystic beliefs. My world has always been firmly anchored in the tangible, the logical. However, in the wake of my mother's passing, something occurred that gently nudged my skepticism aside, if only for a moment.

My mother and I had this playful, albeit slightly irritating, ritual involving the security lock on our front door. Every day, as if by clockwork, she'd leave her bedroom, make sure the main door was locked, and then flip the security handle, leaving it open. It became our little game, one that saw me routinely chiding her for this habit, and her responding with a chuckle, fully aware of the mild annoyance it caused me.

The day after she left us, as I wandered through the house in a grief-filled fog, the weight of her absence pressing down on me, I went to the front porch to read, the routines of daily life moving me forward even as my heart stood still. Upon my return, a sight stopped me in my tracks—the security handle, which I distinctly remember securing that morning after my brother Mick left, was inexplicably flipped open. For a moment, I stood there, bewildered, my mind racing to find a logical explanation. Had I absentmindedly opened it myself? It seemed unlikely, almost impossible, as I had no recollection of approaching the door after securing it.

In that moment, suspended between disbelief and longing, I couldn't help but feel that, in some inexplicable way, it was my mother reaching out. It was as if, in her infinite tenderness and with the mischievous spirit that so defined her, she had found a way to move that latch one last time. To remind me, in the midst of my deepest sorrow, that her presence, her essence, would always linger in the spaces we shared, in the small acts that defined our days together.

I leave the interpretation of this incident open, aware that some may see it as nothing more than a trick of the mind, a grieving son's wishful thinking. Yet, for me, it embodies something profound, a consoling notion that my mother, my best friend, found a way to reach out to me one last time, to partake in our cherished game as a reminder that love—and perhaps the soul—transcends all limitations. It suggests the comforting possibility that she was affirming our previous conversations about the existence of an afterlife. Perhaps she was fine, and would be waiting.

It's a small, personal revelation that I cherish, a subtle sign that in the dance of life and death, love remains, eternally woven into the fabric of our being.

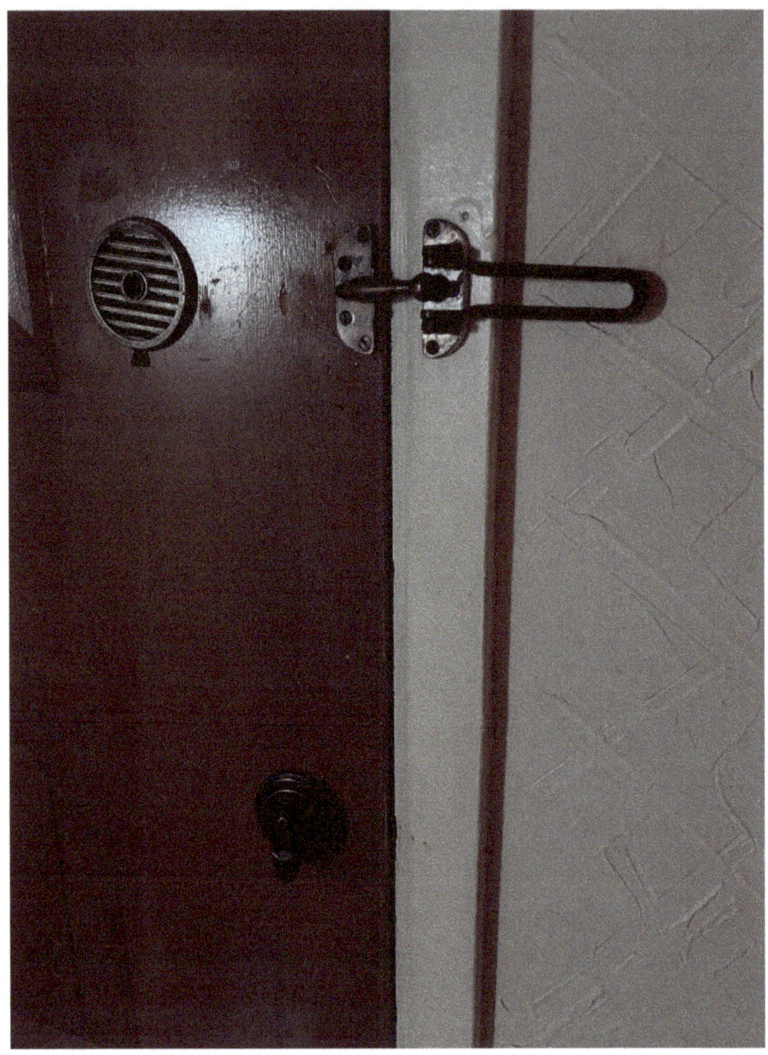

I miss you Mom. Love you more, 3,000 times.

All is Well By Henry Scott-Holland

All is well.
Death is nothing at all.
It does not count.
I have only slipped away into the next room.
Nothing has happened.

Everything remains exactly as it was.
I am I, and you are you,
and the old life that we lived so fondly together is untouched,
unchanged.
Whatever we were to each other, that we are still.

Call me by the old familiar name.
Speak of me in the easy way which you always used.
Put no difference into your tone.
Wear no forced air of solemnity or sorrow.

Laugh as we always laughed at the little jokes that we enjoyed
together.
Play, smile, think of me, pray for me.
Let my name be ever the household word that it always was.
Let it be spoken without an effort, without the ghost of a shadow
upon it.

Life means all that it ever meant.
It is the same as it ever was.
There is absolute and unbroken continuity.
What is this death but a negligible accident?

Why should I be out of mind because I am out of sight?
I am but waiting for you, for an interval,
somewhere very near,
just round the corner.

All is well.

With Thanks

I need to offer gratitude to my entire family, which includes my brothers Mick and Bill, for their instrumental role in enhancing Mom's quality of life in her final years. My sister Marianne played a crucial role in our decision-making process and was a constant beacon of light for Mom. Her unwavering support served as a constant source of strength that kept me going.

I am also thankful to Dr. Steven Massad for his pivotal role as the quarterback of Mom's medical team, and to the EMTs who treated her with utmost care and respect during emergency situations. The dedication of these healthcare professionals and first responders serves as a daily reminder of the true heroes around us.

Additionally, the compassion and expertise of the River Valley Home Health and Hospice team—nurses, physical therapists, memory specialists, and counselors—were invaluable at every stage of Mom's journey. Their dedication, from palliative to end-of-life care, was indispensable in navigating the complexities of her final months. That includes the wonderful and caring Kaisu Fisken, who graciously wrote the Foreword to this book.

Alongside them, I want to express my heartfelt appreciation to all the independent home health professionals who came to our home and cared for Mom. Their tireless commitment to helping the elderly is both inspiring and undervalued in our society. They brought not only their expertise but also their compassion, providing Mom with the dignity and comfort she deserved in her last days. Their presence allowed me to fulfill my role as Mom's caregiver with greater peace of mind, knowing she was in capable hands. To each and every one of them, I am eternally grateful.

Most importantly, thank you Mom and Dad for everything.

-Jim Heath

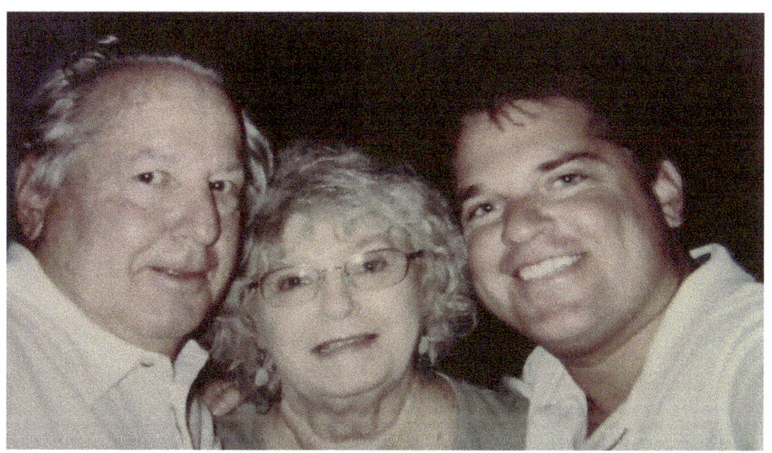

About the Author

Jim Heath, an acclaimed television news anchor, correspondent, author, and political analyst, has carved a remarkable path through the heart of American journalism and political coverage over the past twenty years. His journey from the sunbaked streets of Arizona to the historic landscapes of South Carolina, and finally to the bustling political arena of Ohio, has been marked by 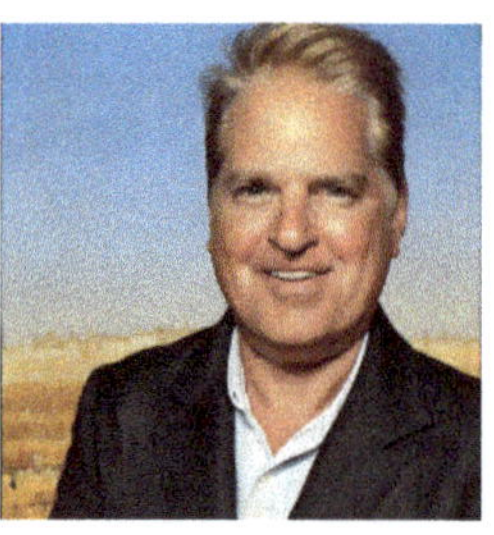 a relentless pursuit of truth and a deep commitment to storytelling.

Heath's contributions to the field of journalism extend beyond the news desk; he is an accomplished documentarian, having written and produced six extensive documentaries focusing on the presidential elections. These works, available on the Jim Heath Channel on YouTube, offer insightful retrospectives on pivotal moments in American political history.

As an author, Jim Heath has reached bestseller status with his book, "Front Row Seat at the Circus: One Journalist's Journey through Two Presidential Elections." This behind-the-scenes exploration offers readers a glimpse into Heath's experiences covering the 2008 and 2012 presidential campaigns. His other notable work, "Covering Mitt," provides a personal account of his interactions with Mitt Romney during the latter's bids for the presidency, reflecting Heath's intimate engagement with the political figures he covers.

Venturing into children's literature, Heath authored "Mylo the Panda," a book aimed at addressing the increasingly negative and confrontational tone prevalent in American discourse. This pivot to children's literature underscores Heath's versatility and commitment to using his voice for positive social impact.

Before his prominence in the media, Heath navigated the corridors of political power as a congressional press secretary and chief of staff to a state Corporation Commissioner, experiences that endowed him with a nuanced understanding of the political process. This background, coupled with his years in precinct politics, has informed his incisive analysis and reporting.

Jim's accolades include the prestigious Walter Cronkite Award for Excellence in Television Political Journalism and two Emmy Awards, highlighting his exceptional contributions to political reporting. His work has also been recognized by the Associated Press and the Ohio Society of Professional Journalists, cementing his status as a respected figure in the field.

Of all his achievements, Jim is most proud to be the youngest son of Rol and Doris Heath.

Resources

The Alzheimer's Association leads the way to end Alzheimer's and all other dementia.

24/7 Helpline: 1-800-272-3900

Online: https://www.alz.org

The National Hospice and Palliative Care Organization enhances and expands access to care that addresses holistic health and the well-being of communities.

Online: https://www.nhpco.org

Help **The American Cancer Society** end cancer as we know it, for everyone.

Online: https://www.cancer.org

The Substance Abuse and Mental Health Services Administration (SAMHSA) provides valuable resources and support for families coping with overwhelming grief.

24/7 Helpline: 1-800-662-HELP (4357)

Online: https://www.samhsa.gov